Theoretical Perspectives for Nursing

Theoretical Perspectives for Nursing

Bonnie Weaver Duldt, R.N., Ph.D.

Professor of Nursing
Assistant Dean of Graduate Programs
School of Nursing
East Carolina University, Greenville, N.C.

Kim Giffin, Ph.D.

Professor Emeritus of Communication Studies
University of Kansas, Lawrence

Little, Brown and Company
Boston   Toronto

Library of Congress Cataloging in Publication Data

Duldt, Bonnie Weaver.
　Theoretical perspectives for nursing.

　Bibliography: p.
　Includes index.
　1. Nursing—Philosophy. I. Giffin, Kim, 1918–
II. Title. [DNLM: 1. Philosophy, Nursing. WY 86 D881t]
RT84.5.D85　1985　　　610.73'01　　　84-28937
ISBN 0-316-19528-6

Library of Congress Catalog Card Number 84-28937

ISBN 0-316-19528-6

9　8　7　6　5　4　3　2　1

MV

Published simultaneously in Canada
by Little, Brown & Company (Canada) Limited

Printed in the United States of America

Acknowledgments begin on page 277.

Preface

In recent years, the nursing profession has started to move away from a topical, subject-oriented approach toward a conceptual and theoretical perspective. Theories of closely related professions and disciplines, such as Maslow's and Erikson's, have been utilized in attempting to understand phenomena observed in human wellness and illness. Since the mid-1960s, nurses themselves have begun to develop theories proposing a systematic view of phenomena observed in the practice of nursing. Such recent nurse-theorists and their theories include Roy's adaptation model, Yura and Walsh's theory of nursing process, and Patterson and Zderad's theory of humanistic nursing. Introductory courses are being formulated in nursing programs to orient students (and practitioners) to one or more of these theories. Nursing educators are using concepts and theories as a basis for curriculum design as well as a framework for content of courses.

We wrote this book for four reasons.

1. A review of current literature reveals few texts whose authors deal with analysis of theories generally, and documentation of how to analyze a nursing theory is rare. Books have been written on development of a theory, such as Dubin's *Theory Building* or Reynold's *Primer in Theory Construction*. But these and other authors are not health professionals. In nursing, a few authors seek to analyze nursing theories at a level so complex that it is too difficult for novices. Their perspective is usually within the discipline of nursing, and frequently they coin words; these characteristics separate aspiring nursing scholars from a communication network intelligible to other disciplines. This book is unique in that we describe the process of theory-building and analysis that is applicable to nursing theories as well as to theories in other disciplines. We use processes of analysis derived from speech communication, rhetorical criticism, and debate. Our perspective is outside the discipline of nursing, looking in. Our terminology is shared by other disciplines, making it easier for the reader to join the communication network among scholars and scientists.

2. Nursing as a discipline is perceived as on the way to becoming a science and a profession. A consensus among scholars seems to be that a theoretical body of knowledge is essential for both a discipline and a profession. Johnson comments on the sparseness of theoretical and scientific giants in nursing's heritage, upon whose work current nursing scholars might build. Consequently, theories and models have been borrowed from other disciplines and professions and applied with varying appropriateness to nursing. Efforts toward achieving knowledge and practice based on theory and research in nursing have occurred only in the past fifteen years.

3. Peer evaluation and accreditation have established criteria and expectations for theory-based nursing education. The National League for Nursing's *Criteria for Appraisal of Baccalaureate and Higher Degree Programs* states that curricula for baccalaureate programs are to be developed within a conceptual framework. Bevis advocates use of theories in curricula to aid both teachers and students "in differentiating the important from the inconsequential in dealing with nursing problems."[1]

4. Nurses have to manage innate and unique barriers as they create theoretical perspectives about nursing. One barrier is the current level of preparation of nursing practitioners. Traditionally, it is expected that development of research and theory will be done by members of a discipline with doctoral-level preparation. We don't have many—currently about two thousand out of more than one million Registered Nurses in the United States. Compared with other disciplines, too large a proportion of our doctorally prepared nurses are not involved in developing or testing theory, and many have limited access to clinical nursing contexts. Therefore we need to have nondoctorally prepared nurses understanding theories and conducting theory-testing research. Another covert barrier is that too many nurses who are involved in research avoid theories. A few minutes flipping through nursing research journals reveals very few articles or research reports that test theoretical statements of relationship, compared to research journals of other academic disciplines. More of our research must test theoretical statements. A third barrier is the historical tendency of nurses to look to medicine or other health-care professions for guidance in developing as a profession and a discipline. We are acutely aware that nursing is derived from many areas of the academic arena, and it seems reasonable that we broaden our perspective and look at the whole academic array of disciplines as we determine our own development as a discipline and a practicing profession. The corrective we suggest is that

1. Em Olivia Bevis, *Curriculum Building in Nursing: A Process*, 2nd ed. (Saint Louis: C. V. Mosby, 1978).

more nurses need to appreciate how important it is to conduct research to test theoretical statements, thus creating a base of scientific and scholarly knowledge for the discipline. Until recently the rank and file of nurse practitioners have not been trained in developing theory or conducting research. Thus theory development at the practice level tends not to occur. Yet it is at this level that relevant phenomena, concepts, and relationships among concepts need to be observed, defined, researched, and implemented as new knowledge. Nursing as a discipline and a profession is at the preconceptual level of development in its theory-building. If our goal is to achieve theory- and research-based nursing practice, then we need to make knowledge about theories and theory testing more easily accessible to all nurses. It is our hope that this book will help achieve this goal.

We aim this book at exerting influence on moving the nursing body of knowledge toward meeting the theoretical criteria of a discipline and a profession. Designed as a text for introductory courses in nursing theories, it is a basis upon which undergraduate and graduate nursing students may develop skills in conceptual thinking and theory development in nursing and a framework for comparative analysis and evaluation of theories. In manuscript form, this book for several years has eased students' way into the mystique of theories, and it reflects their numerous contributions, questions, needs, and feelings.

We have made two assumptions. First, undergraduate students are capable of comprehending and developing theoretical perspectives, and they are currently doing so in disciplines other than nursing. Second, we cannot know which theory or theories will be in vogue over a lifetime of practice; thus, it seems important for nursing faculty to provide a framework for analysis and evaluation of theories generally. As a consequence, future rank-and-file practicing nurses can be equipped with a discriminating and cosmopolitan perspective of theories, nursing-care plans can be based on nursing theories, the incidence of clinical testing of theories will be able to increase, and more of these nurses may seek graduate-level education (formal preparation for conducting research) than current statistics indicate.

This book is divided into four sections. Part One is introductory. In Chapter 1 we set out to establish the need for developing theory in a discipline- and practice-oriented profession such as nursing. In Chapters 2, 3, and 4 we focus on the person as a theorist, particularly in regard to attitudes, use of language, and modes of abstract thinking. In Chapter 5 we discuss generally the building of theories and provide examples of theorists' attitudes, language, and thinking in exploring a phenomenon.

In Part Two we approach a theory as if we were in a biology laboratory and as if a theory were a specimen to be dissected. In Chapter 6 we describe the whole theory or the gross anatomy, and then dissect it into four major parts: the *assumptions, concepts, relationship statements,* and *evaluation.* This is our definition of a theory:

A theory consists of a set of concepts and a set of testable statements relating the concepts within the parameters of a set of assumptions so that a phenomenon is described, explained, predicted, and perhaps controlled.

Following this definition, we identify and define the four major parts of a theory in Chapters 7, 8, 9, and 10. This set of elements serves as an organizing framework for the remainder of the book.

In Part Three the four major parts of a theory are used to establish a method by which one may analyze theories. Chapter 11 consists of a general explanation of the method we propose, and several theories are discussed generally as examples. In Chapter 12 we select Sister C. Roy's theory for analysis as an example of a systems model and we analyze it to demonstrate more fully the method of analysis we advocate. Although this analysis is streamlined and simplified for clarity, it can be much more complex. Our *nursing theory analysis sheets* summarizing Roy's theory are included in the appendixes to help our readers understand this method of grasping the major aspects of any theory and arranging them for comparison with other theories. We believe the method we propose is most helpful in understanding theories and provides a firm basis for comparative theory analysis.

In Part Four we demonstrate how a theory can be developed, using the symbolic interaction model. We present a new theory, Duldt's theory of humanistic nursing communication, share with the profession a first complete statement of this theory, and demonstrate how a theory can be developed from a theorist's perspective. We state the assumptions in Chapter 13, and we discuss how Duldt developed these statements, including sources of influence. Similarly, in Chapters 14 and 15 we present the relevant concepts and relationships. In Chapter 16 we select some representative criteria for evaluating a theory and use these to evaluate the theory of humanistic nursing communication. Our theory analysis sheet (Appendix C) is included to summarize the theory. We believe Part Four will be helpful in "demystifying" theory development for nurses generally and for graduate nursing students in particular.

Finally, in the appendixes, we include theory analysis sheets for other theories that may interest our readers. We propose that you accept the content of these worksheets as a basis for discussion, and we record our perspective on the theory. We encourage you to read the theorist's original documents and develop your own personal and professional opinions about the value of each theory and its potential contribution to your own practice of nursing.

We wish to thank Mary Lou Penney for her assistance in preparing early drafts of the manuscript. We also wish to acknowledge the contribution of many nursing clinicians, students, and faculty who have contributed ideas and examples to this text.

Contents

Theoretical Perspectives for Nursing

ONE

Introduction

It is important that individual students of any discipline or profession, including nursing, achieve early in their careers an orientation to the unique systems of communication that exist among scientists and practitioners in their fields. These communication systems have rules and structures that enable scientists to share a particular view or perspective of those phenomena that are the focus of their discipline. For this reason, knowledge of terminology and thinking processes is analogous to knowledge of a system. Such knowledge is essential for a student's entry into a particular discipline.

In this section, we intend to provide a general structure for learning unique, scholarly communication systems. We establish in Chapter 1 the need for theory development in any discipline or profession. In Chapter 2, the attitude of the individual scholar or practitioner is seen as a significant factor in the development of new knowledge and theory. This individual must also be aware of the need for careful definitions of words or concepts when discussing theory, research, or practice. Thus in Chapter 3 we consider our language and note how easily misunderstandings can occur, hindering the replication of research and the validation of theories.

Chapter 4 deals with a number of ways of thinking used by the various disciplines. Here we also recommend one particular way of abstract thinking for a beginning orientation to nursing. Finally, in Chapter 5, we present an overview of the total theory-building process as it is generally used in nursing and related disciplines. By gaining insight into the structure and process of communication within these disciplines, we hope to provide the reader with an orientation toward and ultimately a sense of inclusion in the unique and scholarly communication systems they encompass.

Why Bother About Theories? 1

We believe that nursing is an important profession and nurses are an important group of professional people who provide a special service for the health care industry. Because of this, we also believe that the field of nursing has a unique body of knowledge.

This body of knowledge comprises a discipline, a set of principles that explain the relationship between what nurses can do and the state of health of their clients. As such, this body of knowledge is constantly growing and changing. New principles are sometimes identified or "discovered." Tentatively held principles are sometimes allowed to become better established. And, occasionally, established principles are abandoned or significantly modified.

For this reason, we believe that nurses need to understand the way in which such principles are suggested, modified, accepted, evaluated, discarded, and established. We believe that professional people, nurses, need to participate in this process, by which the body of knowledge that is fundamental to their profession is refined.

But in order to participate, we have to know how such development takes place. We have to know how nursing principles are discovered and established.

A *set* of related principles is called a theory. Although the word "theory" has more than one meaning, it can be used to refer to a set of related principles, as in such phrases as "a theory of medicine" or "a theory of psychiatry." In this book we will be concerned with a theory of nursing and thus will expect our readers to want to learn how such a theory can be developed, evaluated, modified, improved, and put into practice.

We believe that a properly developed theory of nursing can show that nurses are much more than an extension of the physician, much more than "coordinators" for other health professionals and technicians. We know, of course, that many nurses behave as if they should do only what the doctor tells them to do. For example, if the doctor's orders are that Emily Jones should be given an IV at nine o'clock, then the nurse does just that. However, we believe that the nurse does *not* do "just that." On the contrary, we believe that the way in which the nurse approaches Emily Jones, talks with her, and listens to her, reflects or modifies Emily's emotional state. Thus in addition to applying the appropriate techniques in administering the IV, the nurse's approach itself can contribute to Emily Jones's condition and speed of recovery.

In addition to giving medications, checking vital signs, and recording these and other physical assessment data, the nurse can interact with a client in a very significant way. In fact, the plan of nursing care for individual clients depends on such interactions. But if this principle is to be developed and established in a theory, nurses need to know how such a process is accomplished. They need to know how tentative statements of principles (hypotheses) are stated. They need to be informed about the language of science. They also need to know how hypotheses are tested in a research process and how theories are validated or revised as a result of research findings.

All this is necessary if nurses are to regard themselves as a strong professional group with an established discipline or body of knowledge. The alternative is to regard themselves as technical employees of a hospital, an auxiliary force within the medical profession, or powerless administrative coordinators of professional and nonprofessional health care to individual clients.

From its historical development, it is clear that nursing is achieving the status of a profession and a discipline. For example, Simms states that:

nursing has been in the throes of seeking recognized professional status. In order to do this, nurses must prove that they meet the requirement of society with demands of the profession; i.e., autonomy, distinctive expertness, and control over practice and education.[1]

According to Cohen, this *distinctive expertness* depends on a "theoretical stance which delimits the profession's knowledge base."[2] Since a theoretical stance is a viewpoint or an intellectual attitude, it is clear then that theories are necessary for nursing to be accorded professional status.

In other words, nursing needs a unique body of knowledge that distinguishes it as a separate field of study in the academic world and in society. This is developed by a systematic description of what occurs in nursing and by the generation of many concepts, theories, and models about the field.[3]

Since nursing is unique in that it is both a discipline and a practice-oriented profession, it has an even greater need for a theoretical basis.

For all disciplines, the function of theories is to define, explain, and predict phenomena of each field of study. For example, biology focuses on all life forms and has a classification system for all known animals. Within this discipline, Darwin's theory of evolution seeks to describe and explain how these life forms change, providing the basis by which some persons make predictions about future changes. For practice-oriented professions, however, theories also function as guides to practitioners' actions. In other words, theories need to be prescriptive.[4] For example, the focus of study in psychology is human behavior and emotions. Within this framework, Skinner's stimulus-response theory not only provides description, explanation, and prediction but also serves as a guide to action. Thus the clinical psychologist may choose to use this behaviorist theory to treat an unruly, retarded child. For nursing, the focus of the practitioner's actions is the person having a (wellness or illness) health-care need. In essence, nursing as a practice discipline is "caring," while medicine as a practice discipline focusing on illness is "curing."

The theories practitioners find useful and practical are those that not only serve to describe, explain, and predict but also serve as a guide for practice. Such a prescriptive theory can be defined as that which "conceptualizes both the desired situation and the activities to be used to bring about that desired situation."[5] Generally, prescriptive theories provide some element of control for the practitioner.

Theories for nursing practice have as their major focus four concepts: Man (or human beings), health, society (or environment), and nursing.[6] "Man" is used in the inclusive sense, meaning men and women; sometimes it is also used to indicate the client and the nurse. The goal of nursing generally can be delimited as assisting people in coping with health matters. Thus Newman defines a nursing theory as one that "describes, explains and predicts the patterns of life processes of man which are conducive to health and which prescribe actions to promote these patterns."[7] Such statements also help define the field of nursing.

Historically, some nurses have borrowed relevant theories from other disciplines. However, these theories, according to Wald and Leonard, have failed to provide the guidance required of a theory by a practice-oriented profession and discipline.[8] This is because theories transferred from one discipline to another seem to lose some power in their new context, much as messages lose something in translation from one language to another. For example, Maslow's theory of motivation, particularly his outlining of the set of basic needs, is helpful in assessing a client's health status. However, Maslow's categories are very broad, and nurses have to fill in the details about those basic needs that are relevant to nursing care. In the process, an assumption of Maslow's is violated. He chose to observe superior, performing people whereas in nursing clients often do not meet this criterion because of their health problems. From this it can been seen that nursing theories must be developed by nurses specifically for the context of the nursing practice.

Theories of nursing need to recognize not only the science but also the art of nursing. Indeed, Watson cites numerous leaders in the field, as far back as Florence Nightingale, who have described nursing as being concerned with the subjective, humanistically oriented, and value-centered, yet also organized, objective, and scientific.[9] To be at once concerned with the aesthetic and the scientific is to embrace the yin and the yang, as the Chinese philosophy would state it, of our dualistic world. (See Figure 1.)

Yin and yang, the feminine and masculine, are not sharply separated in such a representation. The curved center line joins the one with the other. And, as if to emphasize the point, in the midst of yin there is the symbolic smaller circle of the yang, and vice versa. The diagram suggests the equality of power and mutual interdependence of these two vast human principles.[10]

Thus methodologies of nursing research need to be congruent with the pathos and the experiential "here and now" of nursing practice as well as with its objective and scientific dimension. This may require the development of our own unique research methodologies to validate nursing theories.

For all these reasons, it is important that nurses know and understand theory analysis and development. As Putt reminds us, "Although it is in varying stages of development, nursing theory does exist and must continue to exist, or else, to paraphrase Pasteur, nurs-

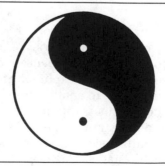

Figure 1. *The yin and yang symbol.*

ing practice will become routines merely born of habit."[11] In other words, theories are necessary to establish nursing as a discipline and as a practice-oriented profession, to define the field of nursing as a scientific arena of study, and to provide guides to action in nursing practice. These are all very important reasons to be concerned about theories.

NOTES

1. S. Simms, "Nursing's Dilemma—The Battle for Role Determination," *Supervisor Nurse* 8 (September 1977): 29–31.
2. Helen A. Cohen, *The Nurse's Quest for a Professional Identity* (Menlo Park, Calif.: Addison-Wesley, 1981), p. 135.
3. Ibid.; Gretchen Crawford, Sister Karin Default, and Ellen Ruby, "Evolving Issues in Theory Development," *Nursing Outlook* 27 (May 1979): 348.
4. Crawford, Default, and Ruby, "Evolving Issues," p. 346.
5. Julia B. George, chairperson, Nursing Theories Conference Group, *Nursing Theories: The Base for Professional Nursing Practice* (Englewood Cliffs, N.J.: Prentice-Hall, 1980), p. 223.
6. Ibid., p. x.
7. Margaret Newman, *Theory Development in Nursing* (Philadelphia: F.A. Davis, 1979), p. 74.
8. F.S. Wald and R.C. Leonard, "Toward Development of Nursing Practice Theory," *Nursing Research* 13 (Fall 1964): 309–313.
9. Jean Watson, "Nursing's Scientific Quest," *Nursing Outlook* 29 (July 1981): 413–416.
10. Patricia Anne Randolph Flynn, ed., *The Healing Continuum: Journies in the Philosophy of Holistic Health* (Bowie, Md.: Robert J. Brady, 1980), p. 262.
11. Arlene M. Putt, *General Systems Theory Applied to Nursing* (Boston: Little, Brown, 1978), p. 7.

The Attitude of a Theory-Builder

It is not easy to maintain the attitude that our hard-earned knowledge—especially our basic principles—cannot be considered as absolute. As we write this book we are constantly aware that we are trying to present fundamental principles by which our readers can look for and assess new information in a way that will provide a solid foundation on which to build and evaluate future theory. The great temptation is to write as if this basic foundation is solid, as if it never changes. But even now we know that some of these principles may need to be changed tomorrow in the light of new discoveries about the way our minds work. Thus, even when we feel most sure and certain of our ground, we also feel the need to maintain an attitude of curiosity about new information, to realize that we must hold basic principles as tentative, expecting change at any time.

All new experiences are perceived in the light of prior ones. In other words, our perception of new information is colored by what we already "know" at the moment. Obviously, interpreting new data by comparing it with relevant data from our earlier experiences, training, and knowledge is a very useful procedure. However, the inherent problem in this tactic arises when we think we know a lot and fail to see new events for what they really are.

In order to accomplish well the steps in the theory-building process, we must have a certain kind of attitude toward the world around us. We must have a deep appreciation of *reliable* principles—ones that are demonstrable, that are supported by evidence and experience, and that stand the test of time. We also must have an inquiring mind—one that is curious, open to new information, and possibly creative or imaginative; one that can live with uncertainty or ambiguity until an issue can be settled by acceptable evidence. In addition, we must have an understanding of the way scholars work together, often competing with one another to gain the first insight into a puzzling set of phenomena (for example, the conditions labeled "arthritis") but at the same

9

time collaborating—sharing information, insights, and reports of research findings. Each of these attitudes will be discussed in this chapter.

THE APPRECIATION OF RELIABLE PRINCIPLES

It can be quite a shock when a child first discovers that an adult may make an untrue statement about the relationship between two or more concepts. This is a "principle" that is *not* a principle. It is a statement that is unreliable; it doesn't work when acted upon.

For many of us this childlike belief in what the "authorities" say carries on into our adult life. Have you ever sat in an airport waiting for the 6:30 flight to be called? Seven o'clock arrives, then 7:30, and you begin to wonder what's going on. Whose word can you depend upon? If the 6:30 flight doesn't leave at 6:30, when will it leave? When is a statement that purports to be a principle one that is reliable?

Unreliable Approaches

Early on in our research for reliable principles we are led to believe that older people (parents) or people with more experience (teachers) or people in charge (authorities) are good sources of principles that work. And for the most part, this is the case. However, at some time in our lives we come to realize that persons in positions of authority are not always in possession of reliable information. They may be misinformed, confused, or dishonest. By the same token, many persons in positions of authority simply adopt the beliefs of those who have held similar positions before them. To a large extent, nothing is so traditional (likely to be believed or acted upon) as tradition. But traditional beliefs can be unworkable, especially in changing circumstances. Thus in the long run we learn that parents, teachers, and other authorities are often sources of dependable principles—but not always.

For ages people have also used insight as the source of their principles. In some cases, such intuitive flashes were excellent hunches, albeit strange and far from the traditional approach. For example, Darwin's "hunch" that one species could "evolve" into another through natural selection is rather famous. However, some scientists are still, after a hundred years, having difficulty accepting the "evolution" of the human "big brain" on the basis of some survival value that would make it naturally selected. It's just too large a change compared with other changes in species' characteristics that are accepted as the result of natural selection. All of which makes a point: the "hunch," to be of real value, must eventually be demonstrably true. If, for instance, the hunch is shown to explain or predict phenomena (such as diseases being caused by bacteria), then it is viewed as very valuable. But if it cannot be proven (such as the belief that flying saucers come from Mars), then it just remains a not very useful possibility.

To be valuable, hunches must be testable. Of course, this is part of the problem with Darwinism and the "big brain." We just don't have a lot of information one way or the other. But with the bacteria example we have been able eventually to test the hunch. Naturally, many hunches have, by definition, been untestable. Most of those attributing various phenomena to the action of spirits are in this category. We just can't get enough information about spirits and their existence to test their alleged influences. Thus when hunches involve some phenomenon that cannot, by definition, be observed (or sensed), they are generally viewed as superstition, as untested notions that are believed by some people who don't fully appreciate the value of a reliable principle and are disbelieved by persons who are more careful.

Sometimes most if not all of us accept unreliable statements or beliefs on the basis of prejudice. How does this work? Prejudice is prejudgment—that is, a judgment made before we have carefully considered the available evidence. Why would a sensible person engage in such behavior? There are many reasons.

Each of us is born into a community, and most of us are also part of a family—a group within a community. In order to get along well with this group and this community, we adopt beliefs, attitudes, and convictions that are similar to those held by the people who surround us. If we are in serious conflict with them regarding norms of behavior and belief then we feel threatened.

When we are small and inexperienced, a personal belief that conflicts with those of people in our family or immediate social group will produce an experience that is somewhat painful. After all, because of this conflict our very basis of existence may be at stake. As we come to identify with our family or with a group in our community we almost inevitably adopt and defend its standards and beliefs. But this identification introduces a degree of narrowness or distortion into our perceptions of the world. We see our group as "us" and persons who are different as "them." In the process, each of us accepts our own distorted perceptions as "reality." Thus customs and attitudes of our reference group are seen by us as superior when they are different from those of foreigners or strangers. Other people and other groups are then judged according to these standards with little regard to their source or validity.

Prejudice is not innate. It is learned behavior, usually arising within a person's family and without conscious intent. As we grow up we are told that "they" are different and have common characteristics and forms of behavior that are inferior to "ours." "They" are believed to be ignorant or immoral or both. Unfortunately, these accepted beliefs provide the basis for stereotypes and prejudices that may last a lifetime.

As the group to which we belong reinforces these beliefs, they are likely to become more intense. When this happens, we as individuals become more willing to express them. And as we give these beliefs our public commitment, they become more deeply ingrained in our thinking. At a later time it will be quite difficult to accept new information or evidence that disturbs these beliefs.

The insular thinking we have just described is a serious barrier to rational consideration of the world around us. There is strong evidence that people of almost all cultures sincerely desire a better world, but they cannot agree as to what constitutes that better world. For the reasons we have described above, members of each culture consider their own group's version of reality and goodness to be fundamentally right. Thus they believe that a better society can only arise from a further elaboration of their own. This is true of Iranians, Hindus, Berbers, Eskimos, Russians, and Americans.[1]

The real difficulty is the *a priori* notion that the ideas, beliefs, or behavior of another person are inferior just because that person is a member of another group or culture. We tend to view such persons as ignorant or evil. This kind of prejudgment—judgment made without taking an open-minded, objective, inquisitive look at the information presented—is properly called prejudice. People of no nation, religion, or group have been entirely free of it.

A particular bias of American culture is to respect the majority opinion. This has come about for good reason—the rejection of the opinion of a powerful minority as the inviolable standard—and it has served us well as a culture wishing to deny the divine right of kings, to resist the powerful influence of the landed gentry, and to deny the tradition of believing persons in authority no matter how they got there. However, a majority can also be selfish, biased, wrong, or even evil. Because of this, the beliefs of minorities need to be considered if a fair approach to the derivation of reliable principles is to be maintained. Minorities can, of course, be equally selfish or in error. But they can also be correct.

Typical Human Behavior

We are now in a position to make some comments about ordinary human behavior as it concerns the determination of reliable principles. At a later point we will contrast this behavior with the approach ordinarily used by scholars, which is frequently called the scientific method.

Ordinary or "average" people generally achieve some confidence in their knowledge of the world by listening, reading, experiencing, comparing, and integrating bits of information from many sources. Very often we call this approach "common sense." In his book *Science and Common Sense*, James Conant has defined common sense as a series of concepts and conceptual schemes satisfactory for the practical uses of mankind.[2] But another famous philosopher, Alfred North Whitehead, has criticized the use of common sense because of its lack of creative thought, calling it a bad master. "Its sole criterion for judgment," Whitehead declared, "is that the new ideas look like old ones."[3] Thus the influence of traditional thinking tends to limit the quality of information usually used by ordinary people.

Typically ordinary persons, employing common sense, are fairly convinced that they know what is true and seek to convince others without carefully considering all possibilities and all available evidence. They do not always start by collecting empirical information based upon careful observations. Quite often they see only what they expect to see, notice the familiar or previously accepted examples or events, and do not fairly consider new or contrary information. Very often they go along with what is believed or accepted by the majority, what most people or "everyone" knows.

The pitfalls we have described above—traditional beliefs, intuition, and prejudice—are constant menaces to the quality of thinking that is often identified as common sense. From time to time they interfere with the accuracy of the beliefs held by ordinary people. However, in many ways ordinary people often think like scientists, carefully observing and analyzing events or experiences before making up their minds. At this point it may be profitable to identify more carefully what we mean by the "method of scientific thinking."

The Method of Science

The basic aim of scientific thinking is one that is common to all of us as ordinary people: to find general understandings and explanations of events in our environment. Scientists seek general explanations that encompass and link together many events and behaviors of things in our world—people, chemicals, and so on. Such general explanations are called theories by scientists. These theories are used by scientists—and sometimes by ordinary people—to understand, predict, and control events around us.

Fred Kerlinger, one of the best-known current writers on the scientific approach, has identified five ways in which scientific thinking differs from common sense. According to him, scientists are said to:

1. Carefully construct a theory (explanation of events), checking it for internal consistency and realizing that it is manmade and subject to possible error.
2. Test hypotheses thus developed against empirical evidence—more than once.
3. Try to control or eliminate the influence of variables, other than those under direct study, as possible "causes" of events.
4. Consciously and systematically try to determine relationships among variables that might be influencing events (outcomes).
5. Rule out "metaphysical" explanations—that is, propositions that by their nature cannot be tested, such as events attributed to "the will of God."[4]

It is quite possible, you may say, that the difference between scientific thinking and the derivation of common sense is more a matter of the degree of careful attention given to important details—developing hypotheses, testing them, making careful observations or measurements, holding beliefs only tentatively, and so on. And perhaps this is true. After all, some people develop uncommonly useful common-sense beliefs. But the fact remains that the *degree of care involved is significant and valuable.* And more important is the fact that some of the five operations we have described appear to be little understood and only poorly used by many people. Perhaps we can understand this difference better if we identify more carefully *what scientists do.*

We already know that scientists develop hypotheses about presumed relationships among natural phenomena; they then test these hypotheses in a systematic, controlled, empirical way. To repeat, *scientists develop only hypotheses that can be tested;* they avoid hypotheses that, by their nature, cannot be tested empirically. In doing so, scientists *order* their investigations so that all possible explanations are considered, using a systematic approach. They *control* their investigations so that all but one causal variable at a time are neutralized or held constant. They seek to obtain *objective* (preferably measurable) data that prove or disprove their hypotheses.

The crucial aspect in the behavior of a scientist is an attitude of curiosity. Because of this, he or she refuses to accept as believable any explanations that have not been carefully stated and empirically tested. Furthermore, the scientist holds all beliefs, even those that have been tested, as tentative explanations, subject to possible revision at any future time. Scientists have inquiring minds. They want to find out why things happen, what causes or influences are involved. They want reliable explanations of the events that occur in their environment.

Scientists usually treat their search for explanations in a problem-solving way. First they seek to find out why something is as it is— why it has certain properties or why certain events transpire. They try to get their "problem" out into the open, make it clear in their minds. Scientists ask why something is, or why something has happened. They try to be as explicit as possible in framing the question they want to ask. Obviously, their use of language is important here, and we'll have more to say about this in the next chapter.

After clearly stating the precise focus of their curiosity, posing the "problem" as it exists, scientists then begin to look for possible answers. They observe related events, conditions, and experiences. They read of the observations made by other scholars. They begin to *formulate hypotheses.* Kerlinger defines a hypothesis as "a conjecture statement, a tentative proposition about two or more observed . . . phenomena or variables."[5] A variable can be any condition that varies. In effect, a scientist says, "I'll bet that if a particular condition occurs (or is arranged) then that other particular condition (or event) will result."

The scientist then *tests* the hypothesis or series of hypotheses. He or she does not test the variables as such; rather, the test is of the hypothesized *relationship* between (or among) particular variables. The scientist measures changes in one variable (the one suspected of being the cause of changes in another) and then measures the changes, if any, in the other variable. By custom, the first or causal variable has come to be called the *independent* variable, possibly because its condition is believed not to be dependent on the condition of the other variable. (This may be a little confusing because the independent variable is often arranged, or changed, by the experimenter.) Not surprisingly, the variable that is suspected of being influenced by the causal variable has come to be called the *dependent* variable, probably because its condition is believed to depend upon the condition of the independent variable.

Setting aside, for the moment, all this terminology, the major point to be understood here is that scientists *test* their hypotheses by measuring observable changes in variables they believe to be related. In other words, *they test the hypothesized relationship* between these variables.

Now we can summarize briefly what scientists do. First, they sense a situation that has not, to their satisfaction, been explained. They try to state specifically what this situation is, treating it as a problem in need of a solution. To do this, they study the relevant literature, the experiences of others, and review their own experience. They then construct a number of carefully stated hypotheses in terms that allow these hypotheses to be tested. Next they test the relationships expressed in these hypotheses and their findings are used in further considerations of the basic situation or "problem," often giving rise to more hypotheses that are then developed and tested. Through this constant activity, the scientific method contributes to our fund of reliable information and helps us to develop useful theories.

THE INQUIRING MIND

In the preceding section we gave some attention to the curiosity of the scientist, to his or her need to know. It is important to look more carefully at the nature of this kind of mind, to explore the mental posture of the scientist.

Curiosity

Scientists have an insatiable desire to seek explanations, to understand how things work and why events happen. When you express one of your beliefs to a scientist, if it isn't clearly stated in terms that are precise or specific, you may get the following response: "Can you restate your belief in terms that can be tested? Can the relationship be measured or at least observed?" In this way, the scientist is seeking to respond only on the basis of empirical data or observations.

But even if your belief is stated in specific, measurable terms, and even if there are data known to support your belief, a scientist will seldom say, "You're absolutely correct." What's wrong with scientists? Why can't they make up their minds?

Open-Mindedness

The subject of open-mindedness has been most carefully studied by the psychologist Milton Rokeach.[6] In fact, he has developed a continuum that extends from absolute closed-mindedness to absolute open-mindedness, depending on the characteristic way in which an individual receives and processes messages from others. On this continuum, the general degree to which a person will change his or her attitude toward an object or concept after learning of another person's attitude toward that same object or concept is the basis of the scale.

Extreme closed-mindedness is identified as "dogmatism." Thus a dogmatic or closed-minded person is described as follows:

1. Likely to evaluate messages on the basis of irrelevant inner drives or arbitrary reinforcements from external authority rather than on the basis of considerations of logic.
2. Primarily seeks information from sources within his or her own belief system. For example, the more closed-minded a Baptist, the more likely it is that he or she will know about Catholicism or Judaism through Baptist sources.
3. Less likely to differentiate among various messages coming from belief systems other than his or her own. For example, an extremely radical rightist may perceive all nonrightists as communist sympathizers.
4. Less likely to distinguish between information and the source of the information and likely to evaluate the message in terms of his or her perceptions of the belief system of the other person.

Essentially the "closed" person is one who rigidly maintains a certain system of beliefs, sees a wide discrepancy between his or her belief system and others that are different, and evaluates messages in terms of the way they fit with his or her own system.

Regardless of their general posture of skepticism regarding a hard-and-fast statement of belief, scientists usually are more open-minded than the average person. They are willing to *consider and investigate* items of new or unusual information. Their curiosity leads them to seek more information, even though they do not readily adopt a firm new belief.

In passing, we must point out that not all noted scientists exhibit at all times the open-mindedness generally associated with the scientific method. There are famous historical examples of the rejection of a new idea by the established authorities—for example, the cases of Galileo on gravity and Darwin on the origin of species—and even today there is far from total accceptance of such discoveries as "Lucy," a skeleton believed to be that of an erect-walking female at least three million years old.[7] Even so, modern scholars generally note such rejection as "bad behavior" on the part of the scientists and uphold the principle of being open to, but careful of accepting, new information and new ideas.

Creativity

Along with an attitude of curiosity and a healthy dose of skepticism, a scientist must be able to engage in creative thought. Throughout our history, scientists have imagined the unimaginable—that microbes smaller than the eye can see could cause smallpox; that a gasoline motor could pull a heavy airplane up into the sky; that the cells in a person's *back* can interpret video signals to the brain as something "seen." (In the last few years scientists have been experimenting with a television camera hooked to an electronic grid strapped to the back of a totally blind person. The grid stimulates cells on the blind person's back according to the degree to which related areas of "view" are picked up by the camera. This stimulation is *interpreted by the brain* as a scene visually experienced *as long as the blind person holds or controls the camera.*[8] The experimenters can't explain everything that is happening, but they are working on it. The point is that they never would have tried the experiment if they could not imagine that a blind person could "see" in this way.)

We don't know as much as we would like to about the process of creative thinking. Having what has been called the "Aha" experience (a flash of brilliant insight: "Aha! I'll bet it's the pressure exerted by the molecules that produces the fusion of the atoms!") is something many scientific researchers have reported. However, to arrange conditions so that you are more likely to have such an experience is a matter that, while under study, is still not well understood. What we suspect happens runs something like this: you must be very knowledgeable in the area about which you are thinking: you must want very much to understand it better; your thinking must be focused on it, but you must be in a relaxed state, willing to divorce yourself from formerly obvious ways of thinking about the topic.[9] We could also suggest that you need a few other characteristics, such as energy, intelligence, and perseverance. These are often suggested if you want to be an inventor. They do seem to be important. However, these three characteristics are also common to many people who are not very creative, people who never have the "Aha" experience. The conditions previously described seem to be the added requirements that make a difference. Even so, at this time, scientists are not really very well informed concerning the required conditions for creativity. But we do know that creativity in the sense of imagining possible new relationships among old patterns of phenomena—the ability to create new, untested hypotheses—is an essential part of the attitude of any scientist who develops a new theory.

Living with Ambiguity

One additional element in the scientific attitude is the ability to tolerate ambiguity. As we find what temporarily appear to be explanations for certain events and conditions, each tentative answer seems to raise many more questions. While this can be frustrating for many of us, scientists have to be able to accept this state of affairs. To be a good scientist, scholar, or theory-builder, we have to learn to live with some ambiguity.

THE COLLABORATION OF SCHOLARS

It is sometimes difficult for young scholars, particularly graduate students searching for a thesis topic, to realize that they must build on the work of other scholars who have gone before them.

Sharing Information

Scientists ordinarily do not take great leaps for mankind without building stairways or platforms bit by bit, brick by brick. A master's thesis may have a brilliant idea, a flash of insight as its major theme. But even so, a reliable theory will have to be built step by step to show the relevance and validity of the brilliant idea.

To accomplish this, scholars must share information, insights, and research results. Their research efforts must be reported carefully and in enough detail so that other scholars can replicate these efforts to determine if they get similar results. You might think that such careful sharing and comparing is more for form than for practical value. And there may be some validity to your criticism when the research topic seems to be of little consequence—such as a comparison of the quality of graffiti on the east coast versus the west. However, think for a moment about the possible treatments we have for cancer. In such areas, we cannot afford to short-change any possible cures, no matter how "unreasonable," and we also need to know for sure if we can take such shortcuts safely. From this we can see that valuable research findings must be shared and tested more than once—in more than one place.

Honesty in Reporting Findings

The need to share research findings and build upon the work of others necessitates honesty in reporting our results. Probably nothing is viewed with such disdain by scholars as dishonesty in this area. Inept thinking is greeted with impatience; lack of clarity is barely tolerated. But outright dishonesty is severely penalized.

In a moment of frustration in the spring of 1974, William Summerlin used a felt-tipped pen to paint a skin graft on a mouse, making a dark, transplanted patch look healthy when it was actually being rejected. When Summerlin's act was discovered, he was dismissed from his appointment to the Sloan-Kettering Institute for Cancer Research in New York. But, interestingly enough, all of his work was not forgotten; indeed, some of his ideas are still being researched by others and appear to be valid and useful.[10] Such are the demands for honesty among scientists that Summerlin had to be exposed and dismissed, but in reports of research by others on his original ideas he is still given credit by those who are continuing his studies.

SUMMARY

The attitudes of scientists are fundamental to the work of theory-building. And central to this process is the appreciation of reliable principles or propositions indicating relationships among variables. In addition, an attitude of perpetual inquiry and collaboration with other scholars is also essential.

In order to discover and establish reliable principles, scientists must refuse to accept beliefs solely on the basis of tradition. To believe something simply because so-called "authorities" believe it is not enough. Instead, scientists must take a look for themselves. Intuitive flashes of insight may be very valuable in this process; they may turn out to be imaginative as well as correct. But scientists must verify their hunches by empirical observation. For this same reason, scientists must guard against prejudice, against forming an opinion without careful consideration of the evidence.

An attitude of constant inquiry, a perpetual need to learn more and obtain answers, involves curiosity, maintaining an open mind toward possible new information or ideas, and the use of creativity in thinking of possible new approaches to old problems. Because reliable answers to many issues are so hard to find, scientists are prepared to live with ambiguity, "knowing" only parts, or making very tentative statements about parts, of the world around us. They are also willing to collaborate with other scholars in sharing information and in honestly reporting the results of their research.

NOTES

1. See a survey of relevant studies by A. W. Combs and D. Snygg, *Individual Behavior*, rev. ed. (New York: Harper & Row, 1959), pp. 341–344.
2. James Conant, *Science and Common Sense* (New Haven: Yale University Press, 1951), pp. 32–33.
3. Alfred North Whitehead, *An Introduction to Mathematics* (New York: Holt, Rinehart and Winston, 1911), p. 157.
4. Fred Kerlinger, *Foundations of Behavioral Research* (New York: Holt, Rinehart and Winston, 1964), pp. 4–6.

5. Ibid., p. 14.
6. Milton Rokeach, *The Open and Closed Mind* (New York: Basic Books, 1960).
7. For a report on the discovery and scientific acceptance of this skeleton, see Donald C. Johanson and Maitland A. Edey, *Lucy: The Beginning of Humankind* (New York: Simon and Schuster, 1981).
8. Richard M. Restak, *The Brain* (New York: Doubleday, 1979), pp. 368–374. Also see Nancy Hechinger, "Seeing Without Eyes," *Science 81* 2 no. 2 (March 1981): 38–43.
9. See Jerome Bruner, "The Conditions of Creativity," in Daniel Goleman and Richard J. Davidson, eds., *Consciousness* (New York: Irvington, 1979), pp. 58–62.
10. Lois Wingerson, "Doing Wrong and Being Right," *Science 81* 2, no. 4 (May 1981): 31–33.

The Language of Science

At the core of theoretical and scientific endeavor lies the human being's unique ability to symbolize. This ability enables us to observe phenomena that are occurring around us; to apply labels or concepts to experiences, events, and happenings; and to place phenomena into conceptual categories. To apply a label is to engage in symbolizing and conceptualizing. This process is applied in science for the purpose of describing, understanding, and predicting—and perhaps controlling—our social and physical environment.

Although human beings share some levels of communication with other living creatures, the abstract ability to symbolize seems to be unique to our species. Of course, many other creatures respond to *signs*. For example, when a horse, a dog, or a human observes the paw print of a bear on a trail, this seems to serve as a sign to all three that a bear has been present and may still be nearby. For humans, the symbol "footprint" is applied to this specific, concrete referent. In a similar manner, most creatures respond to *signals*. When a bell rings, it may be a signal for Pavlov's dog that food is to appear, while for humans a bell may mean that class is over or that someone is calling by telephone. A symbol, "bell," is applied by humans to a scientific referent, the phenomenon of a bell ringing. In contrast, when "*cohesiveness*" happens in a group, or when one person perceives another as being "*trustworthy*," the symbols for these feelings have no concrete referent in reality; thus they are *abstract*.

Unlike animals, humans can be aware of the meaning of a symbol such as "umbrella," even though a real umbrella is not immediately perceived. In short, the human mind can contemplate things that are absent or unseen; this is called *conceptualization*.

ASSIGNING MEANING

An essential element of theory development is the assignment of meaning to specific concepts. Ideally, a concept should mean the same thing to all people, particularly when that concept concerns scientists and theorists. Unfortunately, some other meaning may be assigned unintentionally; this is called *conceptual slippage*. For example, "turkey" generally means a large bird commonly raised on American farms and traditionally served at Thanksgiving dinner. However, "turkey" can also be a label assigned to a member of a group who tends to deviate from accepted social norms; it suggests a cluster of personal characteristics that usually describe someone who is awkward, dumb, disorganized, and undesirable in a rather harmless way.

Sometimes we can be embarrassed when another person ascribes a second meaning to a term. For example, after reaching into a male colleague's desk to get a pencil, a young woman apologetically told him, "Oh, I guess I better ask you first before I reach in your drawers!" Grinning, he quipped, "Honey, you can reach in my drawers any time you want!" Such conceptual slippage can be funny in the social arena, but it can be alarming in others. For example, Secretary of State Haig's announcement, "I am in charge at the White House!" caused quite a stir at the time President Reagan was shot. In the arena of theory and research, it is crucial that concepts be clearly defined so that everyone involved can understand the intended meaning, accept it, and apply it to research and practice. There are a number of ways to achieve this.

First, we may find definitions in *dictionaries*. These references, such as the *American Heritage Dictionary of the English Language*[1] or *Webster's New Collegiate Dictionary*,[2] provide information about how terms or concepts have commonly been used in the past. However, since it often takes three or more years to incorporate new words into our dictionaries, these references cannot be considered current. Definitions tend to be impersonal and to serve as a norm for the use of a particular word in our culture.

Second, one may also look to the *linguistic derivation* or *etymology* of a word; often this is provided in a dictionary and may reveal a new perspective for defining a concept. For example, in attempting to define the concept "anger" for experimental research purposes, the scientific literature seems to present rather confusing, overlapping meanings, and conceptual slippage. The term is often used as if it were synonymous with "hostility," "aggression," and "violence." However, by using a good dictionary Duldt found the following:

Anger is derived from the Latin word, "angere," meaning to strangle or a strong feeling of displeasure about one's throat. In other words, this is an emotion welling up inside one's skin. Hostility comes from the Latin word, "hostilis," meaning to act as if an enemy or to be unfriendly and antagonistic. Aggression is derived from the Latin word, "aggresus," meaning to move toward another for the purpose of attacking or to behave in a destructive manner. Violence derives from the Latin word, "violentus," meaning the tearing of flesh or the act of violating.[3]

Thus through Latin derivations an ancient, orderly progression is found to exist in the meanings assigned to the terms "anger," "hostility," "aggression," and "violence." One marvelous feature of these symbol systems is that they allow us access to the thoughts of our ancestors. And sometimes as in the case of defining "anger," looking carefully at the derivation of the words can be very helpful in clarifying their meanings.

Third, *operationalizing* a concept is yet another way of defining it. What does one do to make a phenomenon happen? Typically, the research reported in the academic journals provides considerable detail when it comes to describing the conditions or equipment necessary to produce a certain phenomenon, such as behavior or a state of being. For example, one group of researchers "operationalized" the degree of hunger that subjects experienced after a period of abstaining from food as the number of crackers and the amount of milk those subjects consumed after a period of starvation. Another group of researchers might "operationalize" hunger by determining the level of blood sugar at varying intervals over time. Still others might simply accept the subject's self-reports to determine when hunger occurs and to what degree. To some extent there is a "leap of faith" between the concept and operationalizing it.

Fourth, a concept is defined by determining what is included or the *scope* of the concept. Closely related, a fifth way is to determine what is excluded or the *limitations*. We can define a concept by drawing a circle to indicate the scope or the abstract territory that concept is to cover. All aspects that seem to reveal the meaning we wish to ascribe to this concept are written or included inside the scope of the circle. Conversely, all meanings we wish to avoid considering appear outside the circle. In this way, let us consider the concept "stress" as defined by Hans Selye.[4] (See Figure 2.) He includes psychological and chemical factors that produce stress reactions in animals and humans, but his definition seems to us to exclude metallic stress and the sort of physical stress that is found in physics and bridge building. It also seems to exclude the stress of particular notes or tones in music and the emphasis of words in inflections, as in speech or linguistics. It has been proposed that as we study concepts we may discover similar scopes and limitations. For example, think of the concept "row," as in rowing a boat or standing in a row or having a row (fight). Generally, the degree of clarity achieved by theorists or researchers in identifying

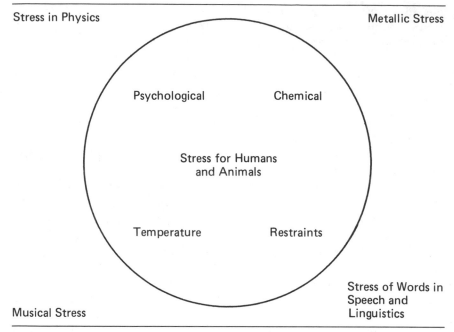

Figure 2. Selye's concept of stress.

the fourth and fifth ways of defining, i.e., inclusions and exclusions of a concept, tends to be associated with the accuracy of interpretation by their colleagues.

A sixth way to define a concept is to state its *role and function* or its *accomplishment.* Ask yourself what function or purpose is served or what goal is reached by the concept. For example, the function of the concept "plumbing" is to transport water. In other words, the conveying of water from one place to another is the action or activity for which plumbing exists. Obviously the role of plumbing has an important effect on our daily habits and expectations: a touch of a faucet provides clean, fresh water at convenient places in our homes, businesses, and the like. We experience considerable inconvenience when something is wrong with the water heater or when pipes freeze, when the plumbing does not perform its role and function as expected. By the same token, if the water becomes contaminated or unsafe, then we can also say the plumbing does not accomplish its purpose or goal.

However, plumbing is a rather concrete and practical example; instead, we need to consider the accomplishment or role and function, of an abstract concept. "Commitment" is a term that is frequently mentioned when we talk about personal relationships. This concept is important because it tends to "accomplish" the binding of people together. It causes us to be loyal to one another, to a group, or to a task goal. When we are committed to someone or something, we promise the resources, skills, or time to help achieve mutually accepted goals. Thus a committed person actively participates and can be depended upon to be there when needed. In other words the role of commitment is to hold people together, to be a social "glue" that is necessary to the foundation of any society. The committed person tends to defend the object of that commitment, whether it is another person, a job, a group, or a country. For example, a major problem America faced during the Vietnam conflict was a lack of commitment to government actions as evidenced by the fact that many people openly demonstrated against the war and left the country to avoid serving in the armed forces.

A seventh way of defining is to provide an *analogy* or a *metaphor*. To use a metaphor is to borrow thoughts, ideas, or contexts to which one symbol may apply so that a new meaning or symbol is developed. In this context, Leonard Hawes identifies three views of metaphors.[5] The *substitution* view involves replacing one symbol for another that is in some way similar. For example, we might say that our brave friend Richard is a lion. The *comparison* view focuses on more specific similarities. Thus, in this view, Richard is like a lion. Finally, the *interaction* view combines two symbols or concepts which interact to give a broader meaning. In the statement, "The poor are the Negroes of Europe," thoughts of the European poor and American blacks interact to produce a unique or different perspective. These are ways in which metaphors expand our symbol system.

Analogies also expand our symbol system by identifying one aspect of similarity between two concepts or entities. For example, the processing of information in the human mind is similar to that of a computer (and vice versa). Obviously, humans and computers differ in most other aspects, but in this one they are alike. According to Hawes, analogies are the basis of theory development.[6] Thus Heider's balance theory is based on the analogy of an old-fashioned scale.[7] Just as the two sides of this scale need to have equal poundage, so Heider proposes that the two sides of human perception must be in balance—that our inside or internal world orientation needs to match our perceived and experienced reality on the outside. In other words, balanced psychological states are preferred, and these states occur when there is perceptual consistency. Another theory based on an analogy is Thibaut and Kelley's theory of interaction outcomes.[8] This theory proposes that the degree of cost or reward that results as an outcome of an interaction between two or more persons tends to determine whether or not the relationship will be maintained. To put it another way, the more positive the "payoffs," the greater the tendency to continue the interaction. This theory seems to be based on the analogy of accounting or economics. Thus, just as a person enters a business venture for the purpose of profits, so Thibaut and Kelley propose that he or she enters an interdependent social interaction for the purpose of maximizing the positive outcome of that participation. We propose that as one considers other theories, one may find other examples of theories based on analogies.

An eighth way to define a concept is to use an *authoritative quotation*, one that reveals descriptive information about the phenomenon itself. Because of this, the person being quoted needs to have immediate, intimate knowledge of and experience with the phenomenon that is being defined. Typically, his or her quotation is taken from a publication, from a book or an article, but excerpts from a speech or impromptu comments noted by a reporter may also serve. Generally, a quotation needs to be germane to the concept being defined, and the person being quoted needs to have some considerable degree of expertise that is widely recognized. Certainly, any quotation needs to be accurate in its content and well documented so that others will be able to refer to the original reference as needed.

Finally, the ninth way to define a concept is by describing a *paradigm* or a *set of elements*. This involves identifying the parts or categories that compose the whole, an approach that is analogous to defining sets in mathematics. Without one part, the set is incomplete. For example, the basic four food groups represent a set of elements for nutrition: breads and cereals, meats and milk, vegetables, and fruits. This is the typical set used to teach clients dietary principles. Another set is typically used to teach nursing students: carbohydrates, proteins, fats, minerals, vitamins, and water. The selection of a set of elements is much like the drawing of a circle around a concept, defining it as one would divide a pie into equal slices. To omit one element would be similar to removing one slice of pie from the whole.

There are two modes of sets: *static* and *process*. The static mode is descriptive and is composed of concepts in the form of nouns. The examples given above regarding sets of elements for nutrition are in the static mode. To cite another example, a static set of elements for human anatomy and physiology, which is commonly used as the basis for organizing chapters in textbooks and modules of courses, includes each of the bodily systems: circulatory, respiratory, gastrointestinal, endocrine, urinary, and so on. In contrast, a process mode requires that the elements are listed in some sequential progression as each realistically occurs and that they are composed of concepts in the form of gerunds (or "ing" words) in order to denote process or change across time. For example, baking a cake consists of assembling (ingredients), measuring, pouring, blending, heating, cooling, and icing.

There are also rules for constructing sets. Generally, the concept (for example, baking) is not repeated as one of its own set of elements; note in the progression above that the term "heating" is used instead. Also, if we develop a set that contains more than about eight elements, we usually review that set to see if two or more of its elements can be consolidated. In addition, the set of elements needs to have a theme or some common factor that denotes cohesiveness. For example, a set of fruit would contain apples, oranges, bananas, pears, lemons, and so on. But a set of apples would not contain oranges. This is the reason the classic medical model (medical, surgical, obstetrical, pediatric, and psychiatric) is no longer advocated by some. It represents a set of mixed elements without a unifying theme. Medicine is an area of practice for a physician; surgery is a method of treatment; obstetrics is concerned with one bodily function of females; pediatrics deals with a particular age group of clients; and psychiatry focuses on one aspect of functioning or behavior. While many programs still follow this classical model, modern curricula in nursing education are organized around sets of elements or concepts according to the levels of adaptation human beings demonstrate in response to stress, to commonly recurring needs during illness, or to the degree to which the state of health is impaired.

LEVELS OF ABSTRACTION

Words or concepts are used to designate varying degrees of abstraction. For this reason, a word may mean one specific representative of a category to one person yet at the same time mean the total category to another. S. I. Hayakawa graphically demonstrates this abstracting effect in his story of "Bessie," the cow.[9] (See Figure 3.)

One way of avoiding or getting into arguments is to move up or down the ladder of abstraction. To move down to specifics tends to intensify an argument, but to move up to higher levels of abstraction is to find some vague generalization upon which both parties can agree. However, the higher the level of abstraction, the greater the ambiguity about the concept's definition and, consequently, the greater the tendency for misunderstandings to occur. The paradox of this is that in theory development we need to conceptualize at a very high level of abstraction, yet at the same time be able to support our conceptualizations by research on specifics. In other words, we need to speak of nurses and clients in terms of nursing theories, yet as we

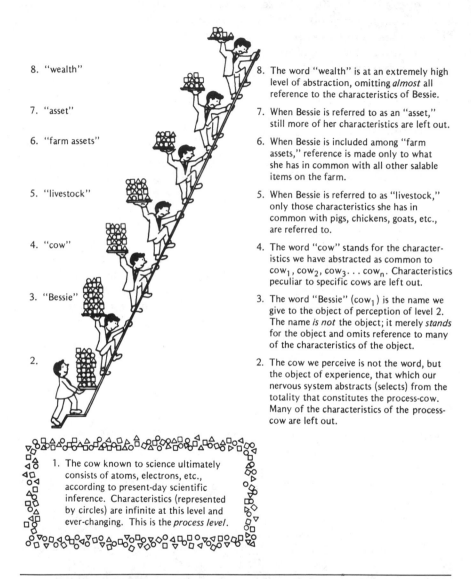

8. "wealth"

8. The word "wealth" is at an extremely high level of abstraction, omitting *almost* all reference to the characteristics of Bessie.

7. "asset"

7. When Bessie is referred to as an "asset," still more of her characteristics are left out.

6. "farm assets"

6. When Bessie is included among "farm assets," reference is made only to what she has in common with all other salable items on the farm.

5. "livestock"

5. When Bessie is referred to as "livestock," only those characteristics she has in common with pigs, chickens, goats, etc., are referred to.

4. "cow"

4. The word "cow" stands for the characteristics we have abstracted as common to cow_1, cow_2, cow_3...cow_n. Characteristics peculiar to specific cows are left out.

3. "Bessie"

3. The word "Bessie" (cow_1) is the name we give to the object of perception of level 2. The name *is not* the object; it merely *stands* for the object and omits reference to many of the characteristics of the object.

2.

2. The cow we perceive is not the word, but the object of experience, that which our nervous system abstracts (selects) from the totality that constitutes the process-cow. Many of the characteristics of the process-cow are left out.

1. The cow known to science ultimately consists of atoms, electrons, etc., according to present-day scientific inference. Characteristics (represented by circles) are infinite at this level and ever-changing. This is the *process level*.

Figure 3. The abstraction ladder. Start reading from the bottom up. (Adapted from "The Abstraction Ladder" in *Language in Thought and Action*, 4th edition, by S. I. Hayakawa, copyright © 1978 by Harcourt Brace Jovanovich, Inc. Reprinted by permission.)

conduct our research, we need to count Mary Jones, R.N., and John Smith with his cerebral vascular accident, or stroke.

Yet another aspect regarding levels of abstraction is that the observations to be made in collecting data about Mary Jones, R.N., and her client, John Smith, may or may not be directly observed. We can check out the reality of physical care provided by Mary Jones, but Mr. Smith's feelings about receiving that care may have to be deduced from his communication behavior. Mr. Smith may express anger about his care, but he may really be angry about his new physical limitations. In addition, the frame of reference of the observer/data collector may differ from that of John Smith and Mary Jones. Mary Jones may expect her client's anger as a natural part of his illness or she may experience her own anger-dismay and avoid going near him. Most people have biases, prejudices, and stereotyped perceptions and expectations concerning stroke victims, and these can impose many other meanings on Mr. Smith's situation. This is true of nurses and even of researchers. While there are tools available to investigate such abstract, unseen concepts, some theorists insist that research data must be observable, and they discredit any research that is based upon unobtrusive methods or the subjects' own reports. This is particularly true of theory and research concepts that have no empirical referent at all, such as the "desire to live" or "therapeutic touch."

SUMMARY

Theoretical conceptualization is concerned with assigning meaning to specific words or concepts. Language is innately a body of generalizations, and misunderstandings about what a word means can easily occur. Thus we have presented a set of nine ways in which theorists and researchers may seek to clarify the assignment of meanings to concepts or categories of phenomena. Yet the very abstractness of concepts is a source of ambiguity that can lead to conceptual slippage. In the next chapter, we will be concerned about how people think with words or concepts in order to make their language work effectively in the development of theories.

NOTES

1. *The American Heritage Dictionary of the English Language*, William Morris, ed. (Boston: American Heritage and Houghton Mifflin, 1969).
2. *Webster's New Collegiate Dictionary*, Henry Bosley Woolf, ed. (Springfield, Mass.: G. & C. Merriam, 1979).

3. Bonnie W. Duldt, "Anger: An Occupational Hazard for Nurses," *Nursing Outlook* 29 (September 1981): 511.
4. Hans Selye, *The Stress of Life* (New York: McGraw-Hill, 1979).
5. Lenord C. Hawes, *Pragmatics of Analoguing: Theory and Model Construction in Communication* (Reading, Mass.: Addison-Wesley, 1975).
6. Ibid.
7. Fritz Heider, *Psychology of Interpersonal Relations* (New York: John Wiley, 1958).
8. J. W. Thibaut and H. H. Kelley, *The Social Psychology of Groups* (New York: John Wiley, 1959).
9. S. I. Hayakawa, *Language in Thought and Action* (New York: Harcourt Brace Jovanovich, 1964), pp. 173–180. Also see Kim Giffin and Bobby Patton, *Fundamentals of Interpersonal Communication* (Harper and Row, 1976), p. 165.

Ways of Thinking

4

Once certain concepts have been defined, members of various disciplines and professions have different ways of thinking abstractly about concepts and formulating theories. While admittedly no small task, merely labeling and describing a phenomenon usually is not enough to understand, make predictions, or control it. These require thinking about how two concepts behave in relation to one another. In this way, principles are developed that can be generally applied to events with some reasonable degree of accuracy.

Some concepts relate to one another so consistently that predictions about future outcomes are relatively simple. For example, when we see dark clouds with lightning and we hear thunder, we know from experience that rain is approaching. We can make this prediction because we understand the relationship between the three concepts—clouds, lightning, and thunder—and because we know they usually combine in such a way that a fourth concept, rain, occurs. Using our knowledge, we can exert some control over the situation by wearing raincoats and using umbrellas.

The simplistic statement we have just explored is one example of a principle drawn from experience. In developing theories, similar relationships are established between concepts, tested and, if verified, stated as principles. A set of such principles makes up the heart of a theory.

DISCIPLINES AND THINKING

Kaplan has identified six ways of thinking or "cognitive styles" of thinking about ways in which concepts relate.[1] Some of these styles have become associated with certain disciplines; the scientists within them use these styles not only to perceive and investigate reality but also to present knowledge.

While most of us develop some degree of proficiency in the use of at least one style of thinking it is important to be aware of and respect other means of expanding knowledge and seeking truth, all of which have merit. Kaplan has labeled these styles literary, academic, eristic, symbolic, postulational, and formal. They are listed here in an order that proceeds from the specific and concrete to the most abstract and content free.

Literary Thinking

Literary style consists of a description of the acts or behavior of an individual or event. This tends to be presented in the form of case studies, autobiographies, or movements in which the acts of individuals or groups are analyzed and interpreted. One example that Kaplan gives is Freud's studies of Moses and Leonardo.[2] Another would be the book *Passages* by Gail Sheehy.[3] The case study approach has long been a popular form of investigation in nursing and other health-related professions.

Academic Thinking

The academic style is a bit more abstract and precise, and according to Kaplan it is verbal rather than operational.[4] In it, ordinary words are used in a special sense in order to constitute a technical vocabulary. Standard idioms in such a vocabulary, together with certain recurrent metaphors, make up a jargon that distinguishes a particular school, a special standpoint or approach to the subject matter.

Academic thinking tends to deal with ideas rather than with observed data, and its treatment of these ideas tends to be highly theoretical, if not purely speculative. Thus ideas are incorporated into a system through the use of great principles that are applied over and over to specific cases, illustrating a particular generalization rather than serving as proof for it.[5] This style is used, for example, in developing categories for historical research or in presenting a sociological analysis of a society.

Eristic Thinking

The eristic style is concerned with debate and argumentation, emphasizing the proof of a proposition, establishment of relationships, and the use of experimental and statistical data. Here a good deal of attention is paid to defining terms, and the scientific method is revered. According to Kaplan, this style of thinking has been the most influential one in the behavioral sciences during this century.[6] Examples of it are plentiful in most journals of psychology and speech.

Symbolic Thinking

The symbolic style is characterized by an artificial language—mathematics. In it, the content is conceptualized in mathematical terms with considerable emphasis on measurement. Through the use of computers and other instruments, such data are processed so that new hypotheses are generated. This style of thinking is commonly found in economics, psychometrics, sociometrics, and game theory.[7]

Postulational Thinking

The postulational style is similar to the symbolic style, but it relies on logic rather than on mathematics. Thus a whole system of propositions or axioms is developed, with the emphasis put on the validity of its proof. This style is frequently used in the behavioral sciences, particularly in the formulation of theories concerning learning, communication, and international relations.

Formal Thinking

The formal style is closely related to the postulational style, but here there is no reference to content. Instead, proof is established by the pattern of relationships that exists among the symbols used. This style of thinking is commonly found in geometry and algebra, and rarely in the behaviorial sciences.

WAYS OF THINKING IN NURSING

We believe the eristic style of abstract thinking is the most applicable and appropriate to nursing. This does not mean, however, that it is the only possible style, or that a nurse cannot use any one of the others. Nevertheless, it has been our observation that most of the basic biological and social sciences traditionally required in nursing curricula tend to use this approach, and that a significant portion of nursing literature appears to be consistent with it. In view of this, it is our judgment that a study of eristic thinking would be most helpful to the beginning nursing student since it would serve as an orientation to thinking about nursing not only as an art and a science but as a discipline and a profession.

The label "eristic" is derived from Eris, the Greek goddess of discord, and it refers to the act of disputing through subtle and specious reasoning. As we mentioned earlier, this style has been developed and applied extensively in the behavioral and social sciences, especially in law and management, social psychology, journalism, and speech. It seems to us that argumentation and debate represents the most characteristic application of eristic thinking. For an in-depth elaboration of this, the reader should consult with such experts as Toulman, Ehninger, and Brockriede,[8] but for our purposes only a brief discussion is necessary.

Eristic thinking involves a set of elements: a claim, a warrant, evidence, reservations, and qualifiers. Each of these elements functions as the organizing particular to more adequately describe the whole, i.e., eristic thinking.

The Claim

A claim is a specific stand regarding an issue. The four types of stands we can take are classified as definitive, designative, evaluative, and activative. A *definitive* stand proposes that something is, was, or will be. For example, we can take a definitive stand by claiming that it is possible to perform an abortion safely. A *designative* stand proposes factual information about the issue. Thus in a designative stand we provide data to indicate that the number of abortions is increasing. An *evaluative* stand proposes the value or worth an issue has had, now has, or will have. Such a stand might state that abortions devalue human life and ruin the moral fiber of our society. An *activative* stand involves policy, an elaboration of what we are to do about an issue. We might, for example, say that a policy of nonparticipation should be established in regard to abortions—in other words, that clients seeking abortions not be admitted to a particular health agency.

Claims may be polarized, pro or con, affirmative or negative. And the four types may also be stated in combinations. For example, we might claim that in accord with humanistic philosophy psychiatric clients must not be put in restraints. This negative stand is both evaluative and activative in that it proposes a humanistic set of values and suggests a policy derived from these values.

The Warrant

The heart of an argument is the warrant, which presents the logical method whereby the claim is established; it responds to the question, "So what?" The warrant is content free and hypothetical. It reveals how we logically move from that claim to the relevant data in order to establish truth. Different types of warrants utilize different types of proof. These are classified as authoritative, motivational, and substantive.

An *authoritative* warrant presents statements or writing by someone who is recognized as an expert on the issue. For example, a well-known psychiatrist might be asked to testify about the previously mentioned claim regarding the restraint of psychiatric clients.

Motivational warrants reveal the reasons we have for wanting the claim, pro or con. For example, humanistic philosophy might be quoted as an example of a motivational warrant for those who want to eliminate restraints for psychiatric patients. And a desire to feel safe or a wish not to be "bothered" or personally involved with the client might be given as a motivating warrant for those wanting to continue the use of restraints.

Substantive warrants include a subset of elements that can be used as a means of proving arguments because they arise from the substance or nature of the issue itself. Generally, these are used in designative stands and concerns about the issue. These include cause and effect, sign, generalization, parallel case, analogy, classification, and statistics.

Cause and effect. If this kind of substantive warrant is used in the restraint issue cited above, then restraints may be identified as the cause of some future effect. For example, if we are arguing negatively, a cause and effect substantive warrant might state that if a person is restrained while he or she is very upset then physical injury tends to result. On the other hand, if we are arguing affirmatively, then we might propose that restraints tend ultimately to have a calming effect on the poor, demented person as limitations of movement come to be accepted.

An effect may also be related to a cause occurring in the past, as lung cancer is commonly related to preceding years of cigarette smoking. Thus in our argument for restraints it might be proposed that the erratic behavior of the client "called for" or caused those nearby to behave in a particular manner—to restrain the client. Because his or her behavior "made us" apply the restraints, we are therefore not responsible. The client is. Or, to argue affirmatively, we might propose that early establishment of interpersonal contact with the client may result in such calmness and relaxation that restraints need not be considered.

Generally, a cause and effect substantive warrant uses information about the issue—that is, the person, event, or condition—and seeks to establish a relationship. "A causes B" is the logical pattern of such thinking. Proofs would involve relating cases or examples in which "A" is shown to have sufficient force to cause "B" to happen.

Signs. A sign substantive warrant indicates that something has occurred. For example, the presence of full milk bottles at the door is a sign that the milkman has been by. Or, to continue our restraint argument, to have a client restrained could be a sign of poor nursing care. However, it may be argued conversely that a restrained patient is a sign of his or her extremely dangerous, assaultive, perhaps even homicidal behavior. "Since B is present, then A must have happened because A is necessary for B to exist" is the logical pattern of this reasoning. In other words, the sign "B" is a symptom of "A." Generally in such warrants additional proofs are not needed. The thing seems to speak for itself.

Generalizations. A generalization is a type of substantive warrant that involves thinking inductively. It proposes that what is true of a few cases in a category tends to be true of all or most. Thus one need only look at a sample to know the whole. "Birds of a feather flock together." This mode argues from the specific to the general. For example, to use such a substantive warrant in our debate about patient restraint, we could cite the restrained patients we have known as representatives to support our affirmative or negative stands. However, this isn't quite as simple as it seems, since there are certain criteria that must be maintained in these kinds of arguments: (a) the instances must be germane to the issue; (b) the sample must be large enough to be homogeneous and representative; (c) the sample must be randomly selected to eliminate bias; and (d) the methods of data collection, measurement, and reporting must be of consistent quality. There seems to be a great tendency in our everyday conversations to ignore the last three criteria as we use our own experiences to "prove" a point.

Parallel cases. A parallel case is a substantive warrant that shows the similarities between two issues to be so strong that they can be considered equal or parallel in nature. The logic in operation here is that "if A causes B in context C_1, then A will cause B in context C_2." For example, we might develop a parallel argument like the following: The initiation of free clinics for drug addicts and intensive anti-drug educational programs in the local schools in a city similar to ours in population and problems reduced the incidence of drug problems among teenagers by 50 percent; thus the initiation of similar clinics and programs in our city may produce similar results. Or, to return to our restraint argument, we might state the benefits or lack of benefits of applying restraints as experienced at the Arkansas State Hospital as support for a stand regarding the use or nonuse of restraints at the Kansas State Hospital.

There is one caution that must be taken in using parallel case arguments: we must be prepared to deal with dissimilarities in the contexts presented. And the greater the number or relevance of these dissimilarities, the less credible the argument. Generally, however, to offer parallel cases is to offer strong support for a particular position.

Analogies. A somewhat weaker substantive warrant, the analogy, must be supported by other forms of proof. We might propose, for example, that just as the staff nurse must keep the head nurse informed about certain task-related events, so the head nurse must keep the nursing supervisor informed about these same events. Of course, there may be numerous differences in the situations of the two individuals; nevertheless in this one respect they are seen as similar. By the same token, in the argument for and against restraints we might state with considerable heat and indignation that to tie up a human being in a straitjacket is just like tying up a dog, and, humanistically speaking, a human being should *not* be treated like a dog. But those speaking in favor of using restraints knowing how dogs are pampered members of some families in our society, might note that humans in mental institutions ought to be treated as *well* as some dogs. Thus it is easy to see how an analogy can be used as supporting proof but not as the bulwark of a particular stand.

Classifications. A classification is a strong substantive warrant in which what is true of a class or total category is proposed as true of any individual representatives of that class or category. This argues from the general to the specific; in other words, it is deductive thinking. The logic is that "A includes B, so if B includes C then A also includes C." Consider, for example, a woman who was expressing concern about a new babysitter. When she discovered that the babysitter happened also to be a nursing student, her concerns vanished. Why? Because of the following proposal: since nursing students tend to be selected by their schools because they are caring, reliable, trustworthy, and conscientious, then this nursing student would tend to have these same characteristics and would probably be a good babysitter.

Using this type of logic in our argument against restraints, it could be proposed that restraints not be used on a particular patient because most patients having the same diagnosis do not need them. Or that since patients requiring straitjackets are totally out of control, and since this patient still responds well to intervention, then he or she does not meet the criteria of the classification for patients needing straitjackets. Although we may have to justify our application of the classification to the particular class member at issue, if we're successful this can be quite a strong argument.

Statistics. The last substantive warrant is a statistical one. In it, numerical relationships are found to exist among raw data derived from specifically designed investigations. These can involve all manner of statistical information from simple counting to descriptive, correlational, and multivariant analysis. Generally, these statistical data are arranged so that they tend to support a particular stand; if they do not support that stand, then they may not be used at all. If necessary we can propose ways in which our opponent's analysis is faulty if there is no strong statistical evidence for our own stand. For example, in our argument regarding restraints, we might cite statistics concerning injuries sustained by patients while restrained—or, conversely, statistics about the number of restrained patients who eventually showed so much improvement that they were discharged, or so little that they are found to be seldom discharged, whichever happens to be true.

In summary, we should remember that any one or more of the substantive warrants we have just discussed may be used either alone or together with the authoritative and motivational warrants to support one of the four types of claim or stand (definitive, designative, evaluative, or activative). With practice and experience, we develop the ability to determine which warrants tend to be the strongest logical basis for our claim. The next step is to provide evidence to substantiate both the claim and the warrant.

Evidence

Evidence provides the issue-relevant content or information that is applied to our logical method. Thus Ehninger and Brockriede define evidence as "an informative statement believed by the listener or reader and employed by an arguer to secure belief in another statement."[9] In other words, the role and function of evidence is to answer the questions, "How do you know?" and "What have you got to go on?"[10] According to Freeley, there are a number of types of evidence: (a) judicial (legal) or extrajudicial; (b) primary (original) or secondary; (c) written or unwritten (oral evidence or artifacts); (d) real (objects) or personal (oral or written testimony); (e) layman or expert (involving special training, knowledge or experience); (f) prearranged (set up by design for proof) or causative (occurring inadvertently with no awareness of its potential future value as evidence); (g) negative (the absence of evidence one would expect to find if the claim were true); and (h) extraneous (evidence that explains or clarifies other evidence). We might choose from these types of evidence to support our claims and warrants about the use of restraints for psychiatric patients. For example, in the parallel case substantive warrant, written evidence in the form of patients' records might be used, as well as clients' personal testimonials of how it feels to be restrained and psychiatric nurses' expert reports. Generally, while a great amount of evidence may be available about an issue, only evidence that is relevant and germane to the issue—and to the claim and warrant—will be useful.

Reservations

In the eristic style of thinking, the reservation provides an escape hatch by limiting the claim to certain conditions or circumstances. It also allows for exceptional cases. While we may wish to make a claim without reservation, its use tends to increase the credibility of our claim. Suppose, for example, it is claimed that psychiatric patients who are restrained struggle against the straitjacket so violently that the skin is bruised and ultimately scarred. This is an absolute statement, implying that such scarring *always* happens. But in fact there may be many instances in which it can be demonstrated that this claim is not true. Thus the proponent of such a claim would indeed have to struggle to maintain his or her position. For this reason, it is generally good practice to include a reservation—an "unless" or an "except for"—in making our claims. Allow for the unusual circumstance. The logical pattern is as follows: "Under unsupervised conditions (C_1), if patients are restrained (A), then struggling (B_1) and scarring (B_2) will occur." (Under C_1, if A, then B_1 and B_2.)

Qualifier

A qualifier functions like a reservation since, according to Freeley, it introduces some "degree of cogency," truthfulness, or credibility.[12] In argumentation, cogency is viewed as a continuum of truth:[13]

Absolute Truth	A Scintilla of Truth

Certainty
...... Probability
.... Plausibility
.... Possibility ......

Certainty is defined as absolute truth. *Probability* refers to the degree of chance that the claim is true. *Plausibility* indicates a fifty-fifty chance that the claim is true. And *possibility* means that the chance of the claim being true is quite unlikely. To complete the continuum, we should also add *incredibility* to indicate the doubtfulness with which the statement is viewed. This continuum can be easily related to theories of probability (*a priori* and *a posteriori*) in statistics.[14]

By adding a qualifier to our previous statement, we now have the following: "Under unsupervised conditions, if patients are restrained, then struggling will tend to occur so that there is a high degree of probability that the skin will become bruised and ultimately scarred." One might even suggest a specific level of probability, such as a statistical probability level of less than five percent. The logical pattern for this is as follows: Under C_1, if A, then B_1 and B_2 with $P < 0.05$. Thus it can be seen that the qualifier provides important information about the degree of truthfulness the proponent attributes to his or her claim. Because of this it may tend to increase the acceptance of the claim by the listener.

So far, we have presented eristic thinking in the framework of argumentation, but we should remember that it is also the basis of both theory development and research in the behavioral and social sciences. The former involves observing a phenomenon and applying a symbol or label to it. This concept is carefully defined so that whenever such a phenomenon occurs it can be detected and measured and consideration given to how this concept relates to other concepts. As a result, a statement may be developed about these two concepts, how each concept works, what they are, and what they do. This is called a principle or a theoretical statement can be made about how the two relate to one another. It is a *claim* and may be restated as a hypothesis, or *warrant*.

Research methods are devised and implemented to gather *evidence*, or data, in order to test a hypothesis or warrant. An analysis of this evidence results in some conclusion regarding the limiting circumstances, or *reservations*, and the probability of truthfulness, or the *qualifier*.

SUMMARY

In order to make the sets and subsets of elements in eristic thinking plain, we can use the following outline:

A. Claim
B. Warrant
    1. Authoritative
    2. Motivational
    3. Substantive
        a) Causes and effects

    b) Signs
    c) Generalizations
    d) Parallel cases
    e) Analogies
    f) Classifications
    g) Statistics
C. Evidence
D. Reservations
E. Qualifiers

The eristic thinking model has important implications for nursing. Since human scientific knowledge is incomplete, that knowledge must be expanded through an elaborate process of theory construction and testing within the scientific community of scholars. Kerlinger summarizes the process in this way:

A Theory is a set of interrelated constructs (concepts), definitions, and propositions that present a systematic view of phenomena by specifying relations among variables, with the purpose of explaining and predicting the phenomena.[15]

This definition assumes the existence of a unique communication system, having rules and structure, that enables scientists to share a "view of phenomena." In most of the disciplines closely related to nursing this communication system is based on an eristic model of thinking.

To have a knowledge of theoretical terminology and thinking processes is to have a knowledge of the rules and structure of the unique communication system that exists among scholars—a knowledge that is essential for inclusion in this communication system. Thus we believe that both nursing students and practicing nurses must be familiar with this system in order to promote their development as professionals and to further the science of nursing as a discipline and a profession.

NOTES

1. Abraham Kaplan, *The Conduct of Inquiry* (Scranton, Pa.: Chandler, 1964).
2. Ibid., p. 259.
3. Gail Sheehy, *Passages* (New York: Dutton, 1977).
4. Kaplan, *Conduct*, p. 259.
5. Ibid., pp. 259–260.
6. Ibid., p. 260.
7. Ibid., pp. 260–261.

8. Stephen Edelston Toulmin, *The Uses of Argument* (New York: Cambridge University Press, 1958); Douglas Ehninger and Wayne Brockriede, *Decisions by Debate* (New York: Dodd, Mead, 1973).
9. Ibid., p. 100.
10. Ibid., p. 101.
11. Austin J. Freeley, *Argumentation and Debate: Rational Decision Making*, 3d ed. (Belmont, Calif.: Wadsworth, 1971).
12. Ibid., pp. 112–115.
13. Ibid., p. 113.
14. Fred N. Kerlinger, *Foundations of Behavioral Research*, 2d ed. (New York: Holt, Rinehart and Winston, 1973).
15. Ibid., p. 9.

The Theory-Building Process: An Overview   5

Scientific thinking is very valuable because it has served our society so well. Indeed, many of our cultural advances appear to be largely the result of scientific thinking. Consider, for example, the improvements in our agriculture, as well as the advances that have brought us autos, airplanes, radios, and television. Consider the data processing we now do by computers, and our great hospitals with their capacity for quick diagnosis and treatment. All these can be traced to scientific thinking.

Of course, there are certain limitations and weaknesses involved in an overadherence to the scientific method. Life would be very dull if we never took a chance, if we never believed in anything until it could be fully tested. And if we're always looking for the causes of things, this can keep us from enjoying those things as they are. Furthermore, if we try to look for one cause for a particular event we can be led into simplistic thinking. There may actually be many factors involved. For example, if your car cannot be started, looking for one single cause of the malfunction may not be enough. There may, in fact, be more than one thing wrong.

It's obvious, then, that scientific thinking can slip up on occasion. But we don't believe such erroneous thinking is really very scientific—and we hope to explain why as we proceed with our study of theory-building.

THE SEARCH FOR PRINCIPLES

At a very early age all of us begin to feel the need for reliable information. Almost without realizing what we are doing we learn the names of things with which we are familiar. Thus, to a large extent, our need for reliable information is oriented toward language and its use.

Concepts

When we see something with which we are unfamiliar we ask, "What is that?" The answer may be, "a bus," or "a train." Whatever it is, the underlying process we are using involves defining *categories* into which we can fit things in our environment. Such categories are called *concepts*.

Gradually we become familiar with concept categories that we can relate to both old and new things: items of clothing such as shoes, socks, dresses, shirts, pants, sweaters, and coats; items of food such as apples, oranges, peas, corn, and spaghetti; items of furniture such as tables, beds, and television sets. We also become acquainted with subcategories such as right shoe and left shoe. In essence, we learn to recognize things as belonging to certain categories; thus we develop a notion of concepts.

Almost any characteristic or set of characteristics may be selected to define a chosen concept. And if a concept is defined so that the special characteristic (or characteristics) can be measured, such a measurable characteristic is often called a *variable* or a dimension, such as I.Q. On the other hand, a concept that can be defined in a speculative way but cannot be directly observed, such as a UFO, is usually called a *construct*. If such constructs become observable at a later time (if, say, we can see hills we thought might be on Mars) they are then viewed as concepts.

Principles

As we grow up we become acquainted with *principles*; these state ways in which concepts are related or fit together. For example, we learn that a "right shoe" goes on our "right foot," a "left shoe" on our "left foot." We learn that a sweater feels awkward if we put it on backwards. Throughout our childhood we spend a lot of time learning such principles: cars are driven on the right-hand side of the street; sidewalks are very hot on summer afternoons; nine times eight equals seventy-two; water is composed of hydrogen and oxygen. And so on. In all this activity we are using language as we describe the relationship between two or more concepts and derive principles.

In the development of theory, concepts are linked together by statements such as "A occurs when B occurs." Scientists view these propositions as tentative until they are demonstrated to be true. In other words, they are identified as *hypotheses*—perhaps true, but in need of testing.

Propositions that link concepts may be of two kinds, related or causal. If A occurs when B occurs, they are said to be related in some way. If in situations where A is great (or in large quantity) B is also great, and where A is small, B is also small, then A and B are said to be *correlated*. On the other hand, if B occurs when A occurs and *only* when A occurs, the A and B are said to be *causally* related. A *causes* B. But if A occurs *only* when B is present then it is inferred that B causes A.

In a later chapter in this book we will have more to say about the value of using language in a very careful way. For the moment, though, we ask only that you realize language's role in helping us to become familiar with concepts and principles.

Why is this important? Because concepts and principles help us get along better in life in two ways. First, they help us understand or explain what is going on around us. They help us reduce the ambiguity and confusion in our surroundings. Second, establishing principles also helps us to predict future events. In these two ways—by explaining our surroundings and by enabling us to predict future events—we learn better ways of enjoying our lives.

Theories

Later on in this book we will carefully define the concept of "theory." However, for now we need only understand that a theory is a *related set of principles*, each principle being a statement that ties two or more concepts together, usually in a correlational or a causal way.

A theory, as a related set of principles, explains phenomena (events, actions, and so on) in a large but identifiable area of investigation or study. Theories help us predict future events within that same area of study.

How do we start to develop useful categories of observed events and behavior that can eventually build a theory? How can practicing nurses contribute to this process? What are the steps involved? In the next section of this chapter we will present an overview of how these questions are answered. Then in later chapters we will study each step in greater detail.

STEPS IN BUILDING A THEORY

Before we proceed to identify and explain the steps in theory-building, there is an overall principle that is so important that we must give it special attention. We think with words. This dependency upon language limits the quality of our thinking: a limited view of the use of language can limit our ability to build theory. This principle is so important that we have devoted an entire chapter to the way in which scientists as theory-builders use words. The need for very careful use of language is inherent in each of the steps in the theory-building process. As we identify these sequential steps, we will be emphasizing in each one the need for clarity and the careful use of words, as well as the inherent difficulties that language imposes on our thinking.

There are four steps in theory-building: identifying our assumptions, defining categories of phenomena (concepts), establishing relationships between or among these categories, and evaluating theories for their practical value in the field to which they may be applied.

Identifying Assumptions

Most of us reach conclusions about the relationships between categories of events or behaviors without realizing that we are relying on assumptions that are often tenuous and sometimes erroneous, such as "The grocery store will have enough money to cash my little paycheck." Usually, it is only when our expectations are not met that we look more carefully at the way we have reached them. In a similar fashion, scholars have learned by frustrating experience that it is valuable to check one's assumptions before proceeding to categorize events, speculate about their relationships, and take a theory out into the practical world.

In fact, many notable advances in our understanding of the world have come about because a theory-builder was forced to reevaluate his or her assumptions. Can we, for example, assume that we can observe all the existing planets? Is there perhaps a tenth planet that's currently invisible? Is it reasonable to assume that all existing viruses have been identified and studied? Should we assume that all cancerous cells behave alike? May we assume that all research is reported honestly?

Assumptions are statements or propositions that are taken to be true. In other words, they are believed not to be in need of further proof or demonstration. For example, we might consider your assumptions about why people need the attention of doctors and nurses. These could include the following:

1. Germs or viruses have attacked their bodies.
2. They have suffered material physical damage, perhaps in an accident.
3. Parts of their bodies have deteriorated or been overtaxed.

You might ask yourself some questions. If indeed some people appear to be ill because of attacks of germs or viruses or because of organic deterioration or overtaxation, how did they get that way? Are you assuming that such things just happen? Or have you made assumptions like the following:

1. They have poor judgment about what their bodies will stand.
2. They have no will to live, perhaps because they believe nobody cares.

If we trace back through the sequence of our assumptions, one thing becomes clear. No matter how clever we are or how sure we are that we know certain principles, our cleverness and assurance rests ultimately on a few basic assumptions, each of which we cannot demonstrate in any realistic way:

1. The world exists.
2. We can discover phenomena in the world through our senses.
3. Phenomena are related in ways other than by chance occurrence alone.

These assumptions are basic to all serious scholarly investigation, but they cannot be "proved" since there is no valid basis for arguing their validity, pro or con. Instead, they are to be recognized for what they are—assumptions. We accept them because we *want* to believe them. That is, they are accepted as true because the alternative is too objectionable to be accepted. And so, armed with these assumptions, we proceed to put observed phenomena into categories and to search for relationships between or among them.

Almost every field of inquiry has a number of further basic assumptions.

1. By experimenting we can determine the cause of (almost) any illness (and thus its cure and care).
2. We can find a cure for a disease without knowing how the cure works—that is, without being able to explain the relevant process in detail.

Probably with a little effort you can think of additional assumptions to add to this list.

Whatever the field in which they operate, it is extremely important that assumptions be stated clearly in the most communicative language possible. And it is even more important that they be clearly identified as we proceed to build a theory. Similarly, in attempting to evaluate someone else's theory we would seek to discern their assumptions; perhaps we will be unwilling to grant these assumptions, and, thus, part or all of the theory will be unacceptable to us. We will look at this issue in more detail later in this book.

Defining Concepts

As we go through the educational process—elementary school, high school, and even college—we often feel the need to use words more carefully, to "look up" precise definitions, to be careful about our choice of language. But our need to define our categories of phenomena (our concepts) is somewhat different when it comes to theory-building. Here the need is to identify or describe a category of phenomena so clearly that we will know immediately (or almost immediately) whether a specific event belongs in or out of a particular category. Perhaps, for example, you think that blonds have more fun. But what does the category "blond" include? Just how dark can blond hair be? And what about "fun"? Does it include getting married? What are we really talking about here?

We know that we are dealing with phenomena—with events, behavior, situations, sets of conditions, almost anything that can be detected directly or indirectly by our senses. But to develop a useful category, we must be able to isolate, distinguish, or "build a fence around" some more or less similar set of phenomena. We must be able to describe the characteristics of phenomena that belong in this category so that any somewhat similar instance will either fit in or out of it. Here, once again, our use of language is extremely important. We must be as careful and precise as possible.

Establishing Relationships

We are here concerned with establishing the existence of relationships between two concepts or among three or more concepts. If there is such a relationship it may be one of two kinds: correlational or causal. As we have seen, in a correlational relationship two or more concepts (categories of phenomena) occur together—concomitantly—and the more of one there is in a given situation, the more there will be of the other. In a causal relationship, one concept produces (or helps to produce) the other. As we determine that two or more concepts are related, we state this in the form of a principle: "A is correlated with B" or "X causes Y." Such statements when put forth tentatively (without proof) are called hypotheses. In other words, they are speculations in need of testing. When testing has occurred and the evidence demonstrates the validity of such statements, we may then call them principles. In some fields, such principles are called theorems or laws, as, for example, in the "law of gravity."

To establish a relationship between or among categories, we must try to make sure that the observed relationship is not a "fluke," that it didn't just happen to occur by chance. However, we might also acknowledge that we can never be absolutely certain about this. We can, though, use safeguards that have grown up by custom among researchers. For example, we can determine that an occurrence is observable in ninety-five out of every hundred similar situations (the "five percent level of confidence"). And in cases where more is at risk, as in a cure for cancer, we may wish to determine if a given relationship may be found in ninety-nine cases out of a hundred or in all but one in a thousand—or one in a hundred thousand. Of course, the amount of our available research resources may limit the certainty with which we can make a claim for a relationship. Thus the application of an uncertain principle will be limited by its potential risk. For example, the use of some drugs for the treatment of alcoholics may be more dangerous than it is advantageous.

As we become able to demonstrate relationships between concepts, thus establishing principles, an additional procedure begins to be possible: the collection of a set of principles into a unified whole—a theory. A theory is a set of principles that, taken together, explain a selected area of investigation.

An Example of Theory-Building

What are the primary ways in which people relate to one another? In answering this question, we could begin by stating that a person tries to satisfy his or her interpersonal needs by establishing relationships with others. In many cases people attempt to build rewarding relationships with whomever happens to be nearby—members of the immediate family, classmates, college roommates, the boy or girl next door. Such relationships appear to be based on convenience; but many times they are not stable or very rewarding. In some cases, the relationship may have started well and brought early signs of interpersonal reward; then, after a time, it became rigid, sterile, and unrewarding. For the most part, however, when we develop our interpersonal relationships we tend to do the best we can, riding out emotional storms, accommodating others whenever possible or when we feel like it, and hoping for the best.

One of the primary goals of many encounter groups is for the participants to take a careful look at themselves and the ways in which they relate to others. When this is done, what are they looking for?

Our interactions are composed of a hundred or more different behaviors; for example, our eyes meet; we smile; we say, "How are you?" Sometimes we act as if we really care. We eat together, work together. We pass one another in the hall or on the sidewalk. We arrange a date to go to lunch or dinner or a movie. On that date we meet, we smile, and so on. Sometimes in working together one of us instructs or supervises the other. We make demands on each other: be on time for our meeting; do this task in this way; be careful with the record-player; don't leave the records on the floor. Sometimes we are tired or lonely and we look for someone who will smile and be friendly while we rest and relax. Sometimes we find someone whose attitudes or thoughts challenge us, lead us along novel or adventurous paths. Sometimes we enjoy being quiet and want others to leave us alone.

Let us say that we find some or almost all of these behaviors in our interactions with most people. How then can we describe a relationship? How can we identify its most important aspects? Are there primary dimensions that matter most? Have these been identified by careful investigation and research? Think back over your interactions with others during the last day or two. What seems to impress you most about the way you and another person get along, about how you relate to each other and feel about each other?

You will probably recall very easily that someone was angry with you or appeared to be. You will also quite readily remember if someone showed you kindness, tenderness, affection—especially if you felt yourself responding in a similar way. Thinking back, you may also find that someone tried to dominate you, demanded that you do something a certain way, tried to "push you around" or "put you down." Or you may, with some thought, remember someone who responded readily to your suggestions, seemed to want your advice, or tried to do things the way you like to see them done.

You may have difficulty recalling someone who seemed to be avoiding you or wanted to be left alone. In fact, they may have been so successful that you did not even notice they were avoiding you. On the other hand, you will likely recall with ease someone who seemed especially interested in talking with you, someone you were with a number of times during the day, a person with whom you interact frequently or for extended periods.

In the two paragraphs above we have suggested that there are different ways of relating to others. But how many of these are really important or significant? Can they be identified and observed in a particular relationship? Can the intensity of each be measured or estimated? If so, we may then be able to characterize a relationship and evaluate it along selected dimensions.

A rather large amount of research tends to support the conclusion that there are three primary dimensions in any human relationship. These are (1) the degree of involvement, (2) the amount of interpersonal control, and (3) the affect or emotional tone (the feelings involved). In his original attempt to identify these dimensions, William Schutz summarized twenty years of research by students of the nature of human relationships.[1] He reviewed sixteen studies of parent-child relations, three analyses of "personality types" of interpersonal behavior, and ten major studies of interpersonal relations in groups. The findings of these studies all converged to support the conclusion that there are three basic dimensions—involvement, control, and affect or emotional tone. Each of these dimensions is different and distinct enough to be measured or estimated. Together they cover the significant elements for describing a relationship. Schutz's own subsequent research has confirmed this conclusion.[2]

The degree of *involvement* in a human relationship refers not only to the amount of interaction between the participants but also to the importance each attaches to this interaction. If two people seldom see or talk to each other—and when they do, they simply exchange impersonal greetings—the degree of their mutual involvement with each other is small. This is especially true if they don't notice that they don't see each other for days. For example, you may have a classmate who ordinarily sits on the opposite side of the room. Did he attend class yesterday? If you can't remember, then your degree of involvement in this relationship is low, even if you tend to see and talk to each other two or three times a week. Conversely, you and your father may live in different cities, may see each other only twice a year and communicate perhaps four or five times a year, and still have a high degree of involvement in your relationship. If each idea your father presents, each sentence he speaks or writes, is given careful thought and attention by you, then your degree of involvement is high.

The degree of involvement between two people is closely related to the amount of personal information they exchange. To be involved with someone, you must know some things about him or her that matter to you, things that are significant.[3] If your involvement with another person is to be high, then you and that other person will have to reveal important parts of yourselves to each other. There are fairly dependable research data showing that when self-disclosure is high, interpersonal involvement is increased.[4]

Suppose, for example, that you meet someone at the tennis courts. You like his looks. This personal information initiates a degree of involvement on your part. You chat for a while and you like the sense of personal values implied by the conversation: he expresses loyalty to his school, regard for his friends, appreciation of personal skill and achievement. You play tennis for an hour and receive impressions of honesty in keeping score, determination to do his best, and fairness in judging out-of-bounds serves. At lunch you are impressed by his courtesy and consideration of others, by the cleanliness of his eating habits, by his friendliness in meeting your needs or wishes. During the next half-hour you hear of his hopes for graduation, his ambition to be a pediatrician, his frustration over the difficulty of certain required courses, and his sadness about the recent loss of a grandfather. If over the ensuing days such self-disclosure continues and you continue to be interested in such personal information, your involvement in the relationship will increase. In addition, his disclosure of the way he feels about you can also lead to your greater involvement.[5] If he shows you the way he feels about your own hopes, ambitions, values, and frustrations, your degree of involvement will be heightened, and the relationship will be of greater importance (especially if it's supportive), both to you and to him.

As people interact and disclose items of personal information to each other, they tend to reach little agreements on what is important and what is not. Out of this sharing comes a working consensus of mutual sympathy and consideration. There is also a tendency to close the gaps between individual differences of opinion. In essence, involvement in a relationship means that the participants interact in ways that are important to each other. And as this involvement is increased, the other two dimensions of a relationship—control and affect or emotional tone—become important. In an established relationship, the degree of involvement is usually quite stable. The amount of interaction may vary from day to day, but these variations are expected and routine. In such a relationship, control and affect are of greatest concern.

In a relationship where involvement has become well established, the primary concerns will thus relate to *control* and *affect*. Interpersonal behavior that is related to control centers on who will make decisions and in what way. Positive control in a relationship is ordinarily referred to as "dominance," "influence," or "rule." This involves the use of power or authority and implies that one person in the relationship assumes the role of superior, supervisor, or leader. Negative control (or lack or control) in a relationship is ordinarily spoken of as "submission," "permissiveness," or "compliance." Here a person is cast in the role of the follower.[6]

Behavior that is related to affect or emotional tone in a relationship involves expressions of warmth, acceptance, and love as well as hostility, rejection, and hate. It is frequently characterized by such positive terms as "friendship," "emotionally close," "sweetheart," and such negative terms as "dislike," "coldness," and "anger."[7]

As we noted earlier, involvement behavior is primarily concerned with the inclusion of another person, with the formation of a relationship. It focuses on the degree of our interaction and our investment of time and energy with another person. Schutz has noted this distinction in the following way: "Basically, inclusion is always concerned with whether or not a relationship exists. Within existent relations, control is the area concerned with who gives orders and makes decisions for whom, whereas affection is concerned with how emotionally close or distant the relation becomes."[8]

The dimension of control may be characterized by a continuum; at one end is *dominance* and at the other is *submission*. The extent to which one person controls the other member of a relationship may be described on a vertical line running between absolute *dominance* and abject *submission* (see Figure 4). In like manner, the dimension of affect or emotional tone may be set on a horizontal axis running between *affection* and *hostility*. Thus the extent to which one person feels affection or hostility toward another in the relationship may be plotted along this horizontal line. Note that each of these basic dimensions of a relationship is bipolar and that each has a "zero" or neutral point in the center.

By way of illustration, your behavior toward another person in a relationship might be highly affectionate or highly hostile or somewhere in between. It might even be neutral —neither affectionate nor

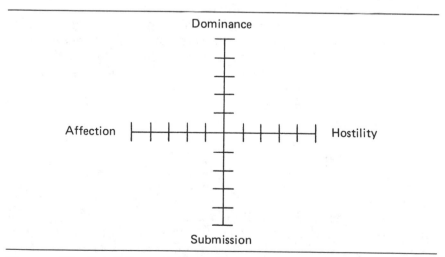

Figure 4. *The D-A-S-H paradigm of interpersonal relationships.*

hostile. In this relationship you might also be very dominant or very submissive or somewhere in between, including neutral—neither dominant nor submissive.

In established relationships, such as those in families or work groups, these two basic dimensions, dominance-submission and affection-hostility, are the primary ones needed to describe the relationship. For example, the most significant aspects of relationships between a father and son, a husband and wife, or a boss and a secretary, can be described on the D-A-S-H paradigm. A large number of fairly sophisticated studies have supported this point.

In one such study, a 1957 investigation that dealt with the relations between psychotherapists and their patients, Timothy Leary and his associates developed a framework for analyzing interpersonal behavior.[9] They identified two major factors; dominance-submission and hate-love. In addition, they represented variations of these elements on a wheel or "circumplex." The four quadrants of the wheel were divided into octants, and eight subcategories were defined. The important thing about this circumplex formulation is that the subcategories were ordered in a circle, without severe breaks or any beginning or end. Thus all interpersonal relationships are included. This formulation has been supported in principle in later studies. Although they used only rough empirical data, the intuition and insight of Leary and his associates seem to be quite remarkable in view of these subsequent findings.

In an early study of mother-child relations, Schaefer identified two major factors: "control-autonomy" and "love-hostility."[10] In a review of other studies of child behavior Schaefer found the same two primary factors; in addition, the primary variables and intervariable relations formed a circumplex.[11] In a study of both mother and father behavior toward children, Slater identified two similar factors: "strictness-permissiveness" and "warmth-coldness."[12] Becker and his associates studied child behavior in relationships with parents and teachers and found two basic factors: "extroversion-introversion" (containing a substantial dominance-submission component) and "emotional stability-instability" (containing a strong hostile-nonhostile component).[13] Following this study, Becker and Krug compared data from six other studies, and two factors emerged: "assertiveness-submissiveness" and "loving-distrusting." Their intervariable correlations also formed a circumplex.[14]

In a series of studies of college students in small problem-solving groups, Borgatta and his associates identified two basic dimensions of member relations: "individual assertivenes" and "sociability." Their relationship variations formed a circumplex.[15] An enlarged follow-up study by Borgatta found similar results,[16] and a rather extensive series of studies of interpersonal behavior of adults by Lorr and McNair also identified two major variables—"dominance-submissiveness" and "affiliation-aggression"—with fifteen intervariable behaviors forming a circumplex.[17]

In 1969, Robert Carson attempted to review all the relevant studies of interpersonal relationships. His survey provided this summary:

On the whole the conclusion seems justified that major portions of the domain of interpersonal behavior can profitably and reasonably accurately be conceived as involving variations on two independent bipolar dimensions. . . . The poles of the second principle dimension are perhaps best approximated by the terms hate versus love.[18]

It is interesting to compare these research findings with the results of scholarship in a related but entirely different area, psycholinguistics, which is concerned with the psychological implications of language usage. A well-known investigator in this field, Roger Brown, made very careful studies of the words used by one person to address another, investigating such practices around the world. Brown concluded that forms of address "are always governed by the same two dimensions: solidarity and status." He noted further that:

Solidarity and status appear to govern much of social life. They lie behind the great regulators of everyday behavior: the way in which similarity generates liking and interaction, which in turn produce more similarity; the way in which differential status confers power and privilege.[19]

There is little question that in essence Brown is referring to the same two basic dimensions of interpersonal relations we have identified earlier: affection-hostility and dominance-submission. Brown concludes that these two factors permeate all human relationships and are obviously important "because we have all had to work them out in order to get along with others."[20]

The lifelong work of Robert Bales should also be viewed in this context. For over twenty-five years, he has been studying interpersonal behavior in various problem-solving or task-oriented groups. In his extensive research he has identified three basic dimensions of interpersonal behavior: "up-down," which is associated with power and conformity; "positive-negative," which is associated with personal liking or group cohesiveness; and "forward-backward," a dimension which is less clearly defined but generally relates to progress in the problem-solving process. Obviously, Bales' first two dimensions are very similar to those in our D-A-S-H paradigm: dominance-submission and affection-hostility. His third category is, we believe, a result of data derived entirely from task-oriented groups. It is reasonable to find in such groups considerable interpersonal behavior relating to progress in using the problem-solving process. This interpretation is in fact suggested by Bales:

> The conceptual scheme of this book associates the forward direction (Forward-Backward Dimension) . . . with task orientation, that is, with task-seriousness. . . . It is assumed that the group to which the system is applied is in a task-oriented phase."[21]

In essence, we believe that Bales' research supports our use of the D-A-S-H paradigm, and further suggests an additional dimension useful in analyzing relationships among members of problem-solving or task-oriented groups.

The theory here was first elaborated by Kim Giffin and Bobby R. Patton in their book *Personal Communication in Human Relations.*[22] The D-A-S-H paradigm can be very valuable as a basic approach in analyzing our own personal relationships since it provides primary dimensions for that analysis. For example, instead of saying to ourselves, "I am usually quite friendly with Bob but he frequently makes me uncomfortable and I get angry," we can use the paradigm to review our relationship with Bob from a broader perspective. In other words, we can ask ourselves where we stand on the continuum of dominance-submission and affection-hostility. Are we generally dominant or submissive? Affectionate or hostile? In this fashion, we can arrive at a fairly comprehensive summary of our relationship. We do this by looking backward and reviewing significant events and behavior in our relationship. In addition, we use the paradigm to observe more carefully the interaction events that occur to us today and in the days to come. We note evidence pro and con our tentative conclusions regarding our relationship. We note especially a friendly smile, our smile unreturned, a warm handclasp, a frown, "hard looks," and other such behaviors (which Erving Goffman calls "tie-signs")[23]—indications that the relationship is generally affectionate or hostile. We also note with greater care any indications that we (or another person) are being dominated, manipulated, influenced, or "pushed around," as suggested by Berne in his book *Games People Play.*[24]

The D-A-S-H paradigm can be very useful in summarizing your relationship with another person. The essential character of any relationship can be graphed on this model. For example, relationships between you (Y) and another person (P) might be summarized in one of the ways shown in Figure 5. Note that the degree of dominance,

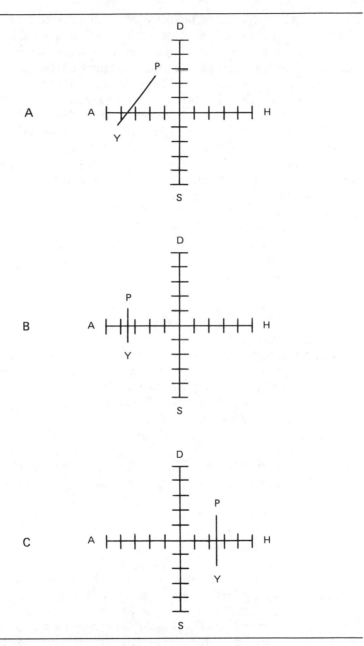

Figure 5. *Examples of possible interpersonal relationships.*

affection, submission, or hostility of each person is shown by the distance of Y or P from the center of the D-A-S-H axes.

As you have been looking over these pages, very likely you have been thinking about one of your own interpersonal relationships. Perhaps it is the one you have with your father. You might conclude, after giving it some thought, that this relationship resembles the one described in Figure 5B. In other words, it involves considerable affection on the part of both of you, but also contains some dominating behavior by your father to which you respond with small tokens of submission. If you are just now entering adult life, it is quite possible that Figure 5C may more accurately describe the current power struggle and attendant emotional feelings between you and your father.

To properly use the D-A-S-H model, you should think carefully about your relationship with another person. Graph it as best you can. Reflect for a while. Compare this relationship with others in which you are currently involved. Also compare it with relationships between other people you know. Review your plot on the graph and change it as seems reasonable. Then pay special attention to events that transpire over a number of days. See if your tentative summary of the relationship seems to be supported. If not, change it to comply with your observations.

As you interact with another person, certain things happen to your relationship that can be explained and to some extent predicted by D-A-S-H paradigm. Let's suppose that you are a young woman and you meet a man you have not met before. As you are introduced and start to get acquainted you find him quite attractive. You also sense that he shows warmth and friendliness, even potential affection. In addition, you note that he tends to dominate your conversation and insists that he take you to lunch. If you stop to think about it, you realize that his interpersonal behavior toward you can be identified as falling somewhere in the dominant-affectionate quadrant. Let us further suppose that your recent experiences with male friends have produced in you a need to resist being led or pushed, and that you are not about to let it happen again, particularly with a new acquaintance. On the other hand, let us suppose that your efforts at resistance of domination have somewhat cooled your relations with other young men, and that at this time you feel warmly appreciative of signs of potential male friendliness and affection.

We can tentatively predict that you and your new acquaintance will engage in a fairly friendly power struggle. In addition, you will be somewhat torn between wanting to accept his friendly attention and resisting his domination. You may, for example, insist on paying for your own lunch but hope he will ask you to dinner. Your power struggle may soon terminate the relationship; either he or you may tire of the required effort and you may not bother with each other further. Or the friendly warmth and potential affection may keep the relationship going; the two of you may find ways of sharing power or influence over each other. Perhaps, for example, you may allow yourself to be dominated only in small ways that do not appear to be very important.

Note that we have said little about where you go together or what you do. You may work together, eat together, exchange personal views and ideas. Of course these things matter. But we are suggesting that what matters most to you in a relationship with another person are the degrees of domination of one over the other and the emotional tone of your feelings toward each other—the degrees of dominance-submission and affection-hostility.

Affection and hostility elicit similar responses. In a relationship affectionate behavior on the part of one person tends to produce an affectionate response on the part of the other. In the same way, hostile behavior tends to produce hostility. Thus behavior that can be characterized as severe hostility nearly always produces resentment, dislike, and anger. Over time, many people learn to hate. We may thus conclude that interpersonal behavior characterized at a certain point along the bipolar dimension of affection-hostility ordinarily elicits a similar response.[25]

Dominance and submission elicit reciprocal responses. Dominant behavior in a relationship tends to produce submissive responses. This is, of course, only true if the interaction continues.[26] If dominant behavior by one person is continued and resistance is shown by the other person, the relationship may very likely be terminated, sometimes before it gets started. If a relationship in which a power struggle occurs is continued, this struggle may last for days, months, or even years. In some families it may never be resolved; it may lead to the use of manipulative games or strategies that continue endlessly.[27] It is interesting to note that while the appetite for sex or comfort is limited, the appetite for power can be limitless.[28]

Submissive behavior in a relationship tends to elicit domination by the other person.[29] Thus if you are dominated, it is not entirely the other person's fault. Submission reinforces dominating behavior, and vice versa. We may thus state a second principle of interpersonal behavior in action: behavior that may be characterized along the bipolar dimension of dominance-submission tends to elicit a reciprocal behavior; dominance reinforces submission; submission reinforces dominance.[30]

Let's turn our attention once again to the imaginary relationship previously discussed: you, a young woman, warmly interacting with a young man who attempts to dominate you in a friendly way. Let us suppose that the interpersonal warmth continues and the attempts to dominate largely subside. The relationship might then be graphed on the D-A-S-H paradigm as illustrated in Figure 6. As you and he interact, your interpersonal behavior as well as his can largely be explained and predicted in terms of the two principles cited above: affection or hostility tend to elicit reciprocal responses. As you and he continue to interact, your behavior produces responses by him; these responses in turn produce responses by you.

The "lock-step" effect. Responses produce responses that produce responses. As you continue to interact with another person, the two of you tend to work out a "shared definition" of your relationship.[31] In some relationships the original "sparring" behavior and early response series may be forgotten; in some cases, it may never have been consciously perceived or noticed; in other cases it may have been misperceived because of anticipated behavior or responses that never actually materialized. However, once the chain of response to response to response behavior has been set in motion, these responses to responses tend to produce what may be called a "lock-step" effect. Once a "lock-step" has become established, it is very diffcult to break. This tendency to respond automatically, almost without thinking, in terms of behavior that is dominant or submissive, affectionate or hostile, is a principle of human relationships identified early by Leary and his associates. Leary called this phenomenon the "interpersonal reflex."[32]

The interpersonal response repertoire. Some people appear to have a narrow or rigid orientation to all or nearly all other people. They tend to respond to nearly all others in about the same way. It's not unusual for this narrow response repertoire to consist of hostile-submissive behavior. Such responses, repeatedly given, tend to elicit a singular hostile-dominant response from others, and thus a rather unsatisfying lock-step goes into full swing.

On the other hand, many persons have a wider repertoire of responses, and can appropriately react in different ways to differing interpersonal behaviors of others. The range of a person's response repertoire tends to determine the degree of rigidity of his or her interpersonal relationships as well as the degree of satisfaction that can be derived from them. Thus a person who relates well with others tends to use a wide range of responses in various different interpersonal situations.[33]

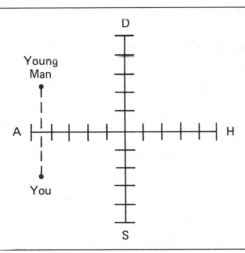

Figure 6. *A warm relationship with a small amount of dominance and submission.*

In contrast, a person with a narrow interpersonal response repertoire is often in trouble. And in cases where one's repertoire is extremely narrow, one's behavior frequently takes the form of showing fear of all people. In ordinary social settings such a person will be notably dysfunctional and will often be identified as "mentally ill."[34]

Less extreme forms of a narrow interpersonal response repertoire very often occur. For example, you may have met "one-way" people who respond to nearly everyone by trying to dominate them while at the same time showing a superficial manipulative friendliness. Such people, of course, are not totally limited in their interpersonal relationships—just narrow in their response repertoire. Another example of a limited repertoire is the "no alternative" person who may say, "I have no alternative but to fire him," or "she left me no alternative." This kind of person often views other people as "things" to be used or manipulated.[35]

On rare occasions two people, each having narrow response repertoires, may succeed in establishing a relationship if the two repertoires are congenial. In this relationship, we can expect to find a very high degree of rigidity and a notable example of "lock-step" behavior.

One of the major purposes of an encounter group or laboratory training group in human relations is to determine the extent of your interpersonal response repertoire. Do you tend to respond in the same way to all group members when they talk to you in different ways? For example, are you always defensive? Do you always act as if people are trying to manipulate or influence you? If some group member shows you friendliness and potential regard or affection, do you show suspicion and hostile resistance? These are very important questions to consider as you attempt to evaluate your ways of relating to others.

We are not always aware of how we are behaving. We actually may be dominating another person when we fully believe that all we are doing is making sure they have sufficient relevant facts. In addition, we are not fully aware of how another person is perceiving our behavior unless he or she gives us adequate verbal or nonverbal feedback. A primary purpose of encounter groups and human relations training is to give us feedback on our interpersonal behavior as it is perceived by others.

In our discussion of a theory of the dimensions of an interpersonal relationship we have illustrated the four requirements that must be observed in collecting a group of related principles to make an integrated set—a theory.

First, from many possibly relevant statements or principles, we search for those that are *basic*. We try to determine the *essential* principles, those that are *required* to explain the phenomena involved. Instead of saying people in a relationship can show courtesy and people in a relationship can show kindness, we search for a larger, more inclusive principle: that people can show positive emotion—warmth, regard, affection.

Second, we search for relevant principles that do not overlap, if at all available. For example, a person who is being *dominant* cannot (at the same time) show *submissiveness*.

Third, we try to develop a *complete* set of principles for our theory—we try to include all principles that are needed to explain the selected grouping of phenomena—not to leave out any that are necessary for our (hopefully) complete understanding of the target area. How we define—set a boundary or "put a fence around"—this selected target area is somewhat arbitrary: it can be as broad or as narrow as we wish an explanation to be. For example, we might want to know how firearms work, or an explanation of the way a recoilless rifle works. What we choose to study, to explain, and thus to theory-build will depend on our interests and on the amount of ambition. Our theory-building can be at a high or low level of abstraction. This fact points once again to the importance of our way of using language.

Finally, we want our theory to include *only those principles that are absolutely necessary* for the understanding of our target area. The principle of parsimony tells us not to allow needless complexity if at all possible. Too many principles can spoil a theory.

In our discussion of a theory of interpersonal relationships we have gone into considerable detail: our purpose was to let you see how a theory is put together—how various principles are selected and what rules apply in an actual theory building operation. You may think we spent too much of your reading time simply to illustrate a process; however, we have a secondary purpose in mind. Later in this book, when we discuss a humanistic theory of nursing, we will be discussing the great importance of nurse-patient relationships. In order to evaluate a relationship we first have to analyze—perceive—its specific dimensions. The theory described in this chapter can provide the basis for just this sort of analysis.

A number of pages back, before we became involved in our illustrative examination of a theory of interpersonal relations, we were describing the steps in theory-building. We have already described three—those involving assumptions, concepts, and the relationships between or among both concepts and principles. Now we will take a look at the fourth.

Evaluating a Theory

To be useful in the advancement of scholarship (or reliable knowledge) a theory must be taken out of the "real world" to see how well it works. If it works well, it will do two things:

1. Explain the relationship among phenomena in the designated area of interest.
2. Predict fairly well the changes in one set of phenomena if changes are made or occur in a related set.

The relationships among a selected set of phenomena (events, behaviors, etc.) are well explained if all *essential* relationships are identified, if they do not *overlap,* if *all* relevant phenomena are explained, and if there *aren't so many details involved that we can't comprehend the theory* in its entirety.

A theory has predictive value if we can show that doing (or changing) A will produce B: will cobalt treatments stop the spread of cancer? If you show hostility toward a doctor, will he show hostility in return?

SUMMARY

In this chapter we have tried to provide an overview of the theory-building process. We started by indicating the value of developing theory in a field such as nursing. We described the way in which all of us search for principles—reliable knowledge with which to make choices, guide our behavior, and live satisfying lives. We described our informal way of searching for concepts (categories of phenomena), principles, and useful theories.

In the latter part of the chapter we described in more detail the formal steps involved in building a theory:

1. Identifying our assumptions.
2. Defining concepts.
3. Establishing relationships among concepts (to develop principles) and among principles (to develop a theory).
4. Evaluating our theories by testing their usefulness in the "real world": do they explain relevant phenomena and accurately predict events or conditions?

In order to accomplish these steps in the theory-building process, we must be aware of four very important factors:

1. We must have a special kind of attitude toward the world around us.
2. We must use language very carefully.
3. We must know what a theory should look like—its essential requirements.
4. We should be capable of analyzing a theory into its relevant parts.

Each of these factors will be treated in a chapter in Part Two. As we go along, we will try to show how each factor has special significance and is essential to the development of a theory of nursing.

NOTES

1. William Shutz, *FIRO: A Three-Dimensional Theory of Interpersonal Behavior* (New York: Holt, Rinehart and Winston, 1958), pp. 34–54.
2. Ibid., pp. 54–56.
3. See Jurgen Ruesch and Gregory Bateson, *Communication: The Social Matrix of Psychiatry* (New York: Norton, 1951), pp. 79–81.
4. See David W. Johnson, ed., *Readings in Humanistic Social Psychology* (Philadelphia: Lippincott, 1972).
5. See David W. Johnson, *Reaching Out* (Englewood Cliffs, N.J.: Prentice-Hall, 1972), pp. 9–10.
6. See Schutz, *FIRO*, pp. 22–23.
7. Ibid., pp. 23–24.
8. Ibid., p. 24.

9. Timothy Leary, *Interpersonal Diagnosis of Personality* (New York: Ronald, 1957).
10. Earl S. Schaefer, "A Circumplex Model for Maternal Behavior," *Journal of Abnormal and Social Psychology* 59 (1959):226–235.
11. Earl S. Schaefer, "Converging Conceptual Models for Maternal Behavior and Child Behavior," in John C. Glidewell, ed., *Parental Attitudes and Child Behavior* (Springfield, Ill.: Charles C Thomas, 1961), pp. 124–146.
12. Phillip E. Slater, "Parent Behavior and the Personality of the Child," *Journal of Genetic Psychology* 101 (1962):53–68.
13. Wesley C. Becker et al., "Relations of Factors Derived from Parent Interview Ratings to Behavior Problems of Five-Year-Olds," *Child Development* 33 (1962):509–553.
14. Wesley C. Becker and Robert S. Krug, "A Circumplex Model for Social Behavior in Children," *Child Development* 35 (1964):371–396.
15. Edgar F. Borgatta, Leonard S. Cottrell, and John M. Mann, "The Spectrum of Individual Interaction Characteristics: An Interdimensional Analysis," *Psychological Reports* 4 (1958):279–319.
16. Edgar F. Borgatta, "Rankings and Self-Assessments: Some Behavioral Characteristics Replication Studies," *Journal of Social Psychology* 52 (1960):297–307.
17. See Maurice Lorr and Douglas M. McNair, "An Interpersonal Behavior Circle," *Journal of Abnormal and Social Psychology* 67 (1963):68–75; Maurice Lorr and Douglas M. McNair, "Expansion of the Interpersonal Behavior Circle," *Journal of Personality and Social Psychology* 2 (1965): 823–830; and Maurice Lorr and Douglas M. McNair, "Methods Relating to Evaluation of Therapeutic Outcome," in Louis A. Gottschalk and Alfred H. Auerback, eds., *Methods of Research in Psychotherapy* (New York: Appleton-Century-Crofts, 1966), pp. 573–594.
18. Robert C. Carson, *Interaction Concepts of Personality* (Chicago: Aldine, 1969), p. 102. See especially Chapter 4, "Varieties of Interpersonal Behavior," pp. 93–121.
19. Roger Brown, *Social Psychology* (New York: Free Press, 1965), pp. 52–53. Also see Roger Brown, *Words and Things* (New York: Free Press, 1958).
20. Brown, *Social Psychology*, pp. 52–53.
21. See Robert F. Bales, *Interaction Process Analysis, A Method for the Study of Small Groups* (Reading, Mass.: Addison-Wesley, 1950); and Robert F. Bales, *Personality and Interpersonal Behavior* (New York: Holt, Rinehart and Winston, 1970), pp. 395–398, 30–50, and especially figs. 3.1, 3.2, and 3.3 on pp. 33–34.
22. Kim Giffin and Bobby R. Patton, *Personal Communication in Human Relations* (Columbus, Ohio: Merrill, 1974), pp. 53–71.
23. See Erving Goffman, *Relations in Public* (New York: Basic Books, 1971), pp. 194–199.
24. Eric Berne, *Games People Play* (New York: Grove, 1964), pp. 91–92.
25. See Leary, *Interpersonal Diagnosis;* also Uriel G. Foa, "Convergences in the Analysis of the Structure of Interpersonal Behavior," *Psychological*

Review 68 (1961):341–353; Uriel G. Foa, "Cross-Cultural Similarity and Differences in Interpersonal Behavior," *Journal of Abnormal and Social Psychology* 60 (1965):517–522; and Uriel G. Foa, "New Developments in Facet Design and Analysis," *Psychological Review* 72 (1965):262–274.

26. See Timothy Leary, "The Theory and Measurement Methodology of Interpersonal Communication," *Psychiatry* 18 (1955):147–161.
27. For a discussion of such tactics and strategies see George R. Bach and Peter Wyden, *The Intimate Enemy* (New York: Morrow, 1968).
28. For a discussion of this principle see Silvano Arieti, *The Will to Be Human* (New York: Quadrangle, 1973), especially Chapter 8.
29. See Leary, "Theory and Measurement Methodology," pp. 155–161.
30. For additional empirical support of this principle see Kenneth Heller, Roger A. Myers, and Linda V. Kline, "Interviewer Behavior as a Function of Standardized Client Roles," *Journal of Consulting Psychology* 27 (1963):117–122
31. See Erving Goffman, *Behavior in Public Places* (New York: Free Press, 1963), p. 96.
32. See Timothy Leary's discussion of "The Interpersonal Reflex" in Leary, "Theory and Measurement Methodology," pp. 153–156. For a critical evaluation of this contribution by Leary, see Carson, *Interaction Concepts of Personality*, pp. 107–115.
33. Leary, "Theory and Measurement Methodology," pp. 152–161.
34. See Carson, *Interaction Concepts of Personality*, pp. 229–232.
35. See the description of the aggressive personality in Karen Horney, *Our Inner Conflicts* (New York: Norton, 1945), pp. 62–72, and the studies of leaders who provide very low value ratings of their co-workers in Fred Fiedler, *A Theory of Leadership Effectiveness* (New York: McGraw-Hill, 1967), pp. 44–46 and 49–59.

TWO

Anatomy of a Theory

One way to investigate a topic is to define it carefully and break it into several parts, analyzing each of those parts in depth. In this section we will investigate the concept "theory" in this manner. In Chapter 6, we explore the definition of theory and identify a set of four major elements that make up the parts of a theory. These elements are further defined in Chapters 7, 8, 9, and 10.

While there are many other ways to analyze a theory, we believe nursing students and others will find the method we propose to be very helpful as an initial approach. Furthermore, we believe this plan is logically consistent with the theoretical perspectives of nursing and of those disciplines that are closely associated with nursing. Thus the information and processes about theories that are learned in these other disciplines will be more readily accessible to our readers.

Defining a Theory

6

In the first part of this book, we proposed that theories are important to disciplines and professions. In connection with this proposition, we considered the attitudes and thinking of scholars and practitioners in theorizing and conceptualizing, and we emphasized the importance of assigning meaning to concepts and defining concepts carefully to avoid misunderstandings.

Since the defining of concepts is viewed as essential to theory development and analysis, it seems appropriate that "theory" as a concept itself be carefully defined. In this chapter, we will do so according to the nine ways to define a concept as outlined in Chapter 3. In addition, each element that is used to build a theory—assumptions, concepts, relationship statements, and evaluation—will also be defined in a similar manner. The concept and set of elements presented in this chapter will then serve as the basis of a plan for the analysis of theories.

DICTIONARY DEFINITIONS, SYNONYMS, AND DERIVATIONS

According to a typical dictionary definition, a theory is "an analysis of a set of facts regarding their relation to one another."[1] This can be described as systematically organized knowledge that is applicable in a wide variety of circumstances. Among the synonyms for "theory" are "judgment," "conclusion," "deduction," "inference," "postulate," "presumption," "assumption," and "presupposition." The Latin derivation is *theoros*, which means to observe or view.

These definitions identify theory in a very general way, but for scientific purposes they do not seem to be specific enough. Since in nursing we are concerned primarily with the behavioral, social, and biological sciences, it seems appropriate, then, to make note of the definitions that are used in these areas. And here Kerlinger's definition seems to be widely accepted:

A theory is a set of interrelated constructs (concepts), definitions and propositions that present a systematic view of phenomena by specifying relations among variables, with the purpose of explaining and predicting the phenomena.[2]

Some definitions of "theory" proposed by scholars in the field of nursing include:

A theory is a set of sentences whose purpose is to explain.[3]

Theory—A way of relating concepts through the use of definitions that assists in developing significant interrelationships to describe or clarify approaches to practice.[4]

Theory is used colloquially to mean an untested idea or an opinion.[5]

A theory is a statement that purports to account for or characterize some phenomenon. A nursing theory, therefore, attempts to describe or explain the phenomenon called nursing.[6]

Nursing theory, then, is theory which describes, explains, and predicts the patterns of the life processes of man which are conducive to health and which prescribe actions to promote these patterns.[7]

For the most part, these definitions seem to be very much like the definitions of an elephant reached in the old fable about the seven blind men. Each man touched a different part of the elephant—the trunk, the tusk, the tail, and so on—and then defined the elephant according to the part he had touched. All were correct insofar as they went, but each was incomplete when it came to defining the whole elephant.

While we are fully aware that we may merely represent yet another blind man defining another part of our theoretical elephant, we would like to propose the following definition:

A theory consists of a set of concepts and a set of testable statements relating the concepts within the parameters of a set of assumptions so that a phenomenon is described, explained, predicted, and perhaps controlled.

We propose this definition not out of disrespect for others' definitions but rather to provide as clearly as we can a basis for understanding and analyzing theories in the manner we advocate.

OPERATIONAL DEFINITION

What must one do to make a theory "happen?" Typically, we read about some event, activity, or thing central to the concern of theorists, the phenomena of a theory. Consider, for example, Maslow's theory of motivation,[8] Erikson's theory of psychosocial behavior,[9] and Skinner's behaviorist theory.[10] All these were presented in writings, but we also hear theories stated. For example, someone might say, "I think what is happening is . . ." or "It seems to me the thing works this way . . . ." Even love stories seem to be based on some idea about how people relate to one another. Theories seem to be all around us. All we need to do is listen for them.

SCOPE

The distinctive ability to think about theories enables human beings to transcend their instinctive responses. We can contemplate symbolically and we can vicariously experience that which may never occur. These abilities are important elements to be included in our theories. Kaplan has identified what he believes to be the necessary components of a theory. According to him, a theory:

1. Involves the use of symbolism.
2. Is related to practice or reality.
3. Remains conjecture until it is validated.
4. Is abstract and conceptual in nature.
5. Explains the truth or certain descriptions of reality.
6. Is necessary to provide its own concepts and generate its own laws or relationship statements.
7. Represents a system of laws or relationships between concepts.[11]

In thinking about these necessary components, we can see that human responses to unfamiliar situations need to transcend habit to create solutions and novel behavior. These new kinds of responses are the behavioral correlates of theory development and thus need to be included in the scope of our definition of a theory.

The concept "theory" includes all symbolic constructions arising from our experiences. However, Reynolds specifies that theories are only those abstract statements that are considered part of scientific knowledge in either a set of laws, or in the axiomatic or causal process forms of theories.[12] Thus his scope for theories seems smaller and more formal. But we believe that the scope for theories in nursing needs to be broader than this in order to assist us in maintaining an open attitude as we look anew at nursing phenomena. Perhaps in time our nursing science will be well enough established to allow formal theory statements.

LIMITATIONS OR EXCLUSIONS

There are several factors that the authorities set outside the boundaries or parameters of a theory. Kaplan, for one, excludes learning by experience:

> To speak loosely, lower animals grasp scientific laws but never rise to the level of scientific theory. They learn *by* experience but not *from* it, for *from* learning requires symbolic constructions which can provide vicarious experience never actually undergone.[13]

Similarly, Reynolds identifies definitions or descriptions of events alone as not constituting a theory. In his view, these merely provide a classification and acknowledge the existence of the phenomenon. He also cites prescriptions for "desirable social behavior or arrangements" as lying outside the realm of a theory.[14]

A third expert, Barbara Stevens, takes the position that "theoryless research," advocated by some in nursing, is really isolated problem-solving. She contends, rather, that every research question comes from some theoretical framework, which simply may not be recognized or stated by the researcher. Stevens further states that the use of one or more theoretical stances for numerous research projects is a most favorable process of establishing the synthesis of a body of knowledge, and she seems to advocate this process for nursing as a discipline and a profession.[15] We support her view.

Often as we study a concept in terms of both its scope and its limitations, we gain a firmer sense of what the concept truly is. It is interesting to note, also, that few authorities speak extensively about what a concept is *not*. For example, none we reviewed mentioned the fact that "theorizing" is not a part of theory development; it refers to casual or idle thought about a subject without consequence.[16]

ACCOMPLISHMENT, ROLE, AND FUNCTION

Kaplan identifies some major accomplishments, roles, and functions of theories.[17] First, theories put things that are known into a system so that (a) we can make sense of otherwise meaningless facts and findings, and (b) we can identify some "rules of the game" so that processes make sense. Second, theories allow a means of verifying truth since hypotheses can be derived from the theoretical statements of relationships and tested so that evidence supports the theory. Third, theories act as guides throughout the research process, particularly in identifying the data to be obtained. Fourth, theories have a heuristic function by serving as tools of instruction. Fifth, theories enhance the growth of knowledge (a) by extension (by defining and exploring fully one small area) and (b) by intension (global exploration of an entire region and then a gradual exploration of the area within that region). Sixth, theories serve to identify questions yet to be answered as well as provide answers for questions we know how to ask.[18]

Usually the purposes of a theory are summarized in definitions and consist of four major functions: descriptive, explanatory, predictive, and prescriptive. Theories describe a phenomenon and explain its processes so that we understand what is occurring. A practical theory will also give information about what will happen or predict outcomes, and perhaps even give directives to guide our actions so we can achieve control of a phenomenon. These, then, are some of the purposes of theories.

ANALOGIES AND METAPHORS

Analogies and metaphors are common in the literature about theories. In fact, Hawes proposes that all theories are based on analogies, and he even uses the term "analoguing" in the title of his book to emphasize the process.[19] Similarly, Kaplan uses the comparison metaphor: as marriage relates two people who are never the same again, so a theory relates two or more concepts that are never again perceived in the same manner.[20]

We suggest that theories are like spotlights on a darkened stage. Just as a beam of light, small in circumference, may reveal a small area of the stage, so some theories are small in scope. For example, the D-A-S-H paradigm gives a perspective of the interpersonal relationship between two people.[21] In contrast, the spotlight may also be wide in circumference and reveal a large area of the stage; and so too a theory may focus on large phenomena. For example, democracy as a theory of political science or government gives a perspective of relationships among people in an entire nation. Just as the intensity of spotlights may vary in the degree of light provided, so theories may vary in the degree of their validity regarding truth and knowledge about our world. It often takes many spotlights of varying size and intensity to reveal the whole of the stage; thus it seems to be most helpful if a discipline and profession has many theories to provide descriptions, explanations, predictions, and perhaps even control over various phenomena.

AUTHORITY QUOTES

In the paragraphs above, we have presented numerous quotations from authorities, particularly in regard to dictionary definitions. Here we would add some definitions from other authorities. For example,

Kaplan states that a theory is "a symbolic construction of a man's creation. Theory is contrasted to experience. Theoretical means abstract, i.e., selects materials from no experience at all."[22]

Shaw and Costanzo propose that "a theory is a convenient way of organizing experiences."[23] And some perceptive graduate student once stated that what we assume leads to the kind of theory we develop—and determines what we will observe. However, this last quotation does not officially "count." We don't remember the person's name and we don't believe this statement was ever published. Thus our source cannot qualify as an expert. Authorities are usually readily available. However, we need to take note of the degree of credibility that can be attributed to them before we accept their quotations as worthy of our careful consideration.

SET OF ELEMENTS

Some authorities have set up classification systems to categorize theories according to a particular theme. In this connection, Kaplan speaks of two types of theories, concatenated and hierarchical.[24] A *concatenated* theory explains facts and laws by placing them within a pattern. Examples of this type of theory include the "big bang" theory of the origins of the universe, Darwin's theory of evolution, and Freud's psychoanalytic theory. In contrast, *hierarchical* theory is a pyramid of deductions. The base of the pyramid consists of *facts* from which *initial conclusions* are derived, and which in turn can be summarized into *premises*. These premises lead to sets of basic *principles* and ultimately to general *laws*. A model of a hierarchical theory may be viewed as a pyramid of deductions, as seen in Figure 7. This type of theory is typically used in postulational and formal styles of thinking, which are common to the disciplines of mathematics and calculus. Among examples of hierarchical theories are the theory of relativity, the theory of Mendelian genetics, and the theory of Keynesian economics.[25]

Another classification of theories that Kaplan describes is based on content rather than form. Thus each theory is viewed as having an "explanatory shell" which draws a line around the phenomena that are viewed by the theory. In this way, the theory is seen as an "isolated system" that specifies "things necessary and sufficient for an explanation . . . of the event in question."[26] We may, then, have *macro* or *molar* theories and *micro* or *molecular* theories according to the circumference of the explanatory shell. In economics, for example, we may have a macrotheory that deals with the economy of an industry

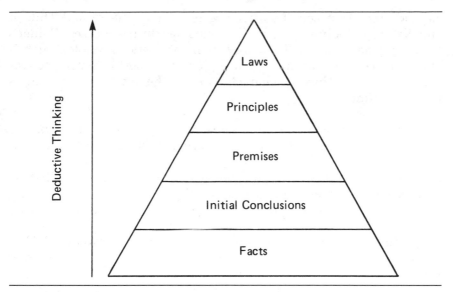

Figure 7. Pyramid of deductions.

or a country; we may also have microtheories that focus on the ways in which one person functions economically.[27]

Another way to classify theories is according to the degree to which they break with current perspectives or the degree of uniqueness of the theorist's idea or paradigm. A paradigm (which is derived from the Latin word *paradigma*, meaning to show side by side)[28] consists of diagrams, graphs, and verbal outlines the theorist uses to show concepts and the relationships among them.[29]

Kuhn identifies a set of three such levels of paradigms.[30] The first is the "Kuhn paradigm," which represents the theorist's greatest break with past and current perspectives. Examples include Columbus' theory that the world is round, Darwin's theory of evolution, and Freud's theory of personality. The characteristics of the Kuhn paradigm are summarized by Reynolds as follows:

1. It represents a radically new conceptualization of the phenomena.
2. It suggests a new research strategy or methodological procedure for gathering empirical evidence to support the paradigm.
3. It tends to suggest new problems for solution.
4. Application of the new paradigm frequently explains what previous paradigms were unable to explain.[31]

The second level is the "paradigm," which consists of a new orientation but is somewhat similar to other ideas. Examples of this include

Heider's theory of cognitive balance or balance theory and Thibaut and Kelley's theory of interaction outcomes. In these cases, Heider's theory is analogous to the theory of homeostatic physiological balance, and Thibaut and Kelley's theory draws on cost-gain perspectives from economics. Thus the characteristics of the paradigm are summarized as follows:

1. The conceptualization represents a unique description of the phenomena, but a dramatic new orientation or "world view" is absent.
2. Although new research strategies may be suggested, dramatic new procedures or methodologies are absent.
3. The new conceptualization may suggest new research questions.[32]

The third level Kuhn identifies is the "paradigm variation." This level includes theories that add details or refinements to another theory but do not alter our basic perspective of the phenomena. An example of this type would be Newcomb's ABX theory of Communicative Acts, which develops details of Heider's balance theory. In addition, the work of Adler, Jung, and others can be described as paradigm variations of Freud's theory of psychoanalysis.[33]

Theories are also classified according to levels of complexity by Dickoff and James.[34] They identify four levels, the first of which is "naming theory" or factor isolating theory. This is the lowest level of theory construction in which concepts of the phenomena are labeled and described. The second level is "factor relating" theory. At this level, the described concepts are associated in a relationship statement. The third level is "situation-relating" or explanatory theory. It is at this level that hypotheses can be developed that predict events. The fourth level is "situation producing" or prescriptive theory, which suggests actions that are required to reach desired situations.

There are many additional ways to categorize information about theories for pedagogical purposes. We propose the following four process elements as another helpful one:

Assuming

Assuming is a process in which we first perceive some phenomenon, event, or occurrence that presents itself in reality and wonder how it happens. For example, Maslow's theory focuses on human behavior and seeks to answer the question, "Why do people behave the way they do?"[35] In this process, certain factual or descriptive statements or assumptions are presumed to be true and are not tested. For example,

Maslow presumes or assumes that humans function as integrated wholes rather than in parts.

Conceptualizing

Here the phenomenon is assigned a term, a word, or a concept that is then defined and described for the theory. This definition is made very carefully so that all will easily be able to identify the phenomenon and the concept as belonging together. Maslow, for example, identified the phenomenon of his theory and labeled it with the concept "motivation." He then developed a set of elements according to needs. He used needs as the theme of this set since he assumed that human needs are the power or force of motivation.

Relating

Within the framework of the assumptions, the manner in which the concepts are associated or changed is clearly described in formal statements of relationship, in propositions, or in claims. This represents the heart of the theory and is necessary to meet Kerlinger's definitional criteria of a theory—that is, that it explains and predicts phenomena.[36] One relationship statement Maslow makes is that a person's lower-level needs must be met to a considerable extent before his or her awareness of higher needs becomes salient.

Evaluating

Finally hypotheses are derived from the relationship statements, tests and experiments are conducted, and data are analyzed and interpreted. Ultimately some judgment is made regarding how truthful, valid, reliable, and believable the results are—and, ultimately, the degree to which these results support the theory. The research support for Maslow's theory of human motivation has been massive, so that the theory has influenced many disciplines, nursing in particular. Maslow's set of basic needs is often used as a check list to verify the completeness of planning for nursing care of both individuals and groups of clients.

SUMMARY

We have presented a systematic and extensive definition of the concept "theory" according to the nine ways of defining a concept. We have also proposed a set of four elements for a theory: assuming, conceptualizing, relating, and evaluating. In the next four chapters, each of these process elements will be discussed as a separate part of the whole, as if they were systems of the human body to be studied one after another. In addition, each element will be discussed according to the nine ways of defining a concept.

NOTES

1. *Webster's New Collegiate Dictionary*, Henry Bosley Woolf, ed. (Springfield, Mass.: G. & C. Merriam, 1979), p. 1200.
2. Fred N. Kerlinger, *Foundations of Behavioral Research*, 2nd ed. (New York: Holt, Rinehart and Winston, 1973), p. 9.
3. Sister Callista Roy and Sharon L. Roberts, *Theory Construction in Nursing: An Adaptation Model* (Englewood Cliffs, N.J.: Prentice-Hall, 1981), p. 2.
4. Julia B. George, ed., *Nursing Theories: The Base for Professional Nursing Practice* (Englewood Cliffs, N.J.: Prentice-Hall, 1980), p. 224.
5. Dorothea E. Orem, *Concept Formulization in Nursing: Process and Product* (Boston: Little, Brown, 1979), p. 55.
6. Barbara J. Stevens, *Nursing Theory: Analysis, Application, Evaluation* (Boston: Little, Brown, 1979), p. 1.
7. Margaret Newman, *Theory Development in Nursing* (Philadelphia: F. A. Davis, 1979), p. 74.
8. Abraham H. Maslow, *Motivation and Personality* (New York: Harper and Brothers, 1954).
9. Erik H. Erikson, *Childhood and Society* (New York: W.W. Norton, 1950).
10. B. F. Skinner, *Science and Human Behavior* (New York: Macmillan, 1953)
11. Abraham Kaplan, *The Conduct of Inquiry* (Scranton, Pa.: Chandler, 1964), pp. 294–298.
12. Paul Davidson Reynolds, *A Primer in Theory Construction* (Indianapolis: Bobbs-Merrill, 1971), p. 11.
13. Kaplan, *Inquiry*, p. 295.
14. Reynolds, *A Primer*, p. 11.
15. Stevens, *Nursing Theory*, pp. 184–185.
16. *Webster's Dictionary*, pp. 1109, 1200.
17. Kaplan, *Inquiry*, pp. 302–326.
18. Ibid.
19. Leonard C. Hawes, *Pragmatics of Analoguing: Theory and Model Construction in Communication* (Reading, Mass.: Addison-Wesley, 1975), p. ix.
20. Kaplan, *Inquiry*, p. 297.
21. See the discussion of the D-A-S-H paradigm in Chapter 5. Also see Kim Giffin and Bobby R. Patton, *Personal Communication in Human Relations* (Columbus, Ohio: Merrill, 1974), pp. 53–71; and Bonnie W. Duldt, "Sexual Harassment in Nursing," *Nursing Outlook* 30 (June, 1981):336–342.
22. Kaplan, *Inquiry*, pp. 295–298.

23. Marvin E. Shaw and Philip R. Costanzo, *Theories of Social Psychology* (New York: McGraw-Hill, 1970), p. 9.
24. Kaplan, *Inquiry*, pp. 298–299.
25. Ibid.
26. Ibid., p. 299.
27. Ibid., pp. 299–300.
28. *Webster's Dictionary*, p. 823.
29. Kerlinger, *Foundations*, pp. 134, 300.
30. Thomas S. Kuhn, *The Structure of Scientific Revolution* (Chicago: University of Chicago Press, 1962).
31. Reynolds, *A Primer*, p. 22.
32. Ibid., p. 26.
33. Ibid., pp. 21–43.
34. J. Dickoff and P. James, "A Theory of Theories—A Position Paper," *Nursing Research* 17 (1968):197–203; J. Dickoff and P. James, "Researching Research's Role in Theory Development," *Nursing Research* 17 (1968):204–206. Also published in Catherine C. H. Seaman and Phyllis J. Verhonick, *Research Methods for Undergraduate Students in Nursing*, 2nd ed. (New York: Appleton-Century-Crofts, 1982), pp. 126–127.
35. Maslow, *Motivation*.
36. Kerlinger, *Foundations*, p. 9.

Assumptions 7

The first sequential element in the process of developing a theory is assuming. We make assumptions daily. Suppose, for example, that you and a friend are enjoying a pleasant conversation over coffee when a loud, unfamiliar noise is heard. You and your friend would probably look at one another and then glance about. One of you would probably ask, "What was that?" The conversation thereafter would focus on information about the unfamiliar noise, formulating assumptions and hunches about what caused it. "It's just thunder," "The boiler must have exploded," or "Mom just drove into the garage door again!" may be some of the conclusions you might reach. All of these comments are based on assumptions made about the situation.

Often we are not aware that we are making assumptions. But when we think about it, it's obvious that assuming is of practical value in our daily lives, as well as a vital element of theory development. In this chapter, we will give careful consideration to the concept "assuming" and define it according to the nine ways of defining a concept.

DICTIONARY DEFINITIONS, SYNONYMS, AND DERIVATIONS

An assumption is a given, an assertion that supposes a thing to be true. It is a proposition, axiom, postulate, or notion that has been assumed. "To assume" means to arbitrarily or tentatively accept that something is true. It is taken as a premise, as in logic. In other words, a statement is accepted or supposed to be true without proof or demonstration. Synonyms for "assumption" include "presupposition," "postulate," "posit," "presumption," and "premise." The Latin derivation is from the term *assumere*, meaning to take, to consume.[1]

Moving from this general definition to the area of specific disciplines, we find more precise definitions. For example, as a behavioral scientist, Kaplan states that theorists make assumptions about the solution or about the "problematic situation" itself.[2] And in the nursing literature, Stevens states that nurse theorists need to state assumptions about the situation or "context" in which nursing takes place: "Often it must be inferred from unstated assumptions; thus one may find that the context on which a theory is built is that of an ill person in a hospital setting."[3] Generally, nursing authors tend to define assumptions as statements that are accepted as true without testing.[4]

OPERATIONAL DEFINITION

Making assumptions is a process in which we observe a particular phenomenon, wonder about how it happens, and develop some hunches. Kaplan calls these hunches "presuppositions," explaining that "we draw our presuppositions from earlier inquiries, from other sciences, from everyday knowledge, from the experiences of conflict and frustration which motivated our inquiry, from habit and tradition, from who knows where."[5] In this process, we start from what we know or believe about the phenomenon. These beliefs or presuppositions are our own assumptions, our perceptual window through which we view the phenomenon and all the data that are relevant to it. Changes in these presuppositions are, according to Kaplan, rare and represent a scientific revolution.[6] Examples of such revolutions include changing our belief that the sun revolves around the earth in favor of the belief that the earth revolves around the sun, believing that the earth is round rather than flat, and believing that diseases are caused by an ecologically based, interaction process instead of simply by germs. The process of observing, wondering about how things happen, and developing presuppositions results in the generation of such assumptions.

Examples of the assumptions we make can easily be found in our daily lives. In the Judeo-Christian religions, the Bible is usually assumed to be the word of God; this is accepted on "faith," and is not questioned by those who believe. Once something is accepted as a valid assumption, one's behavior probably changes accordingly. We assume, for instance, that the driver of another car will stop for the red light at an intersection. We even assume that the light is in fact red from the other driver's perspective. As nurses, we often assume that the physician has written the correct dosage in ordering a medication. We assume that the equipment packaged in plastic containers is sterile. It is only when we question and investigate our assumptions that they are no longer assumptions. At this point, they are restated as relationship statements or hypotheses. We can note when this happens, because our behavior tends to change as our assumptions switch to hypotheses and become the focus of our investigations and examination.

Generally, however, our assumptions "happen" daily, and it is common for us to accept them without even stating them. But in theory development assumptions are formally stated and thus are helpful in communicating the specific perspectives of the theorist.

SCOPE

Obviously we make assumptions about a wide variety of subjects. The following is a sample of the topics about which some well-known theorists have made assumptions in the course of their work:

1. What is the goal and nature of science? Is Man to control or to coordinate the world?
2. What is the nature of human beings? Are humans good, bad, or neutral? Are humans merely reactive to the environment about them or can they be proactive, initiating changes through choice?
3. What is the nature of human motivation? Is it based on needs, as proposed by Maslow,[7] on self-concept as posited by Schutz,[8] on goal attainment as assumed by Skinner,[9] or on cognitive development as proposed by Piaget?[10]
4. What is the nature of truth? How do we know reality? What does reality include? Does it consist only of what can be seen, as the behaviorists contend, or does it also include self-reported experiences and awareness, as contended by the humanists? Does it also include extrasensory perception (ESP), precognition, and other awarenesses reported by spiritualists and psychics?
5. Is one's past an influence on one's behavior as proposed by "trait" theories? Or is one to consider only the present situation as posited by the "state" theories?
6. What is the appropriate level of analysis for a theory? Should a theorist consider only individual elements or should groups and entire species be considered? Should cells be the level of analysis or should one consider entire societies?

The choices made among these approaches clearly influence a theorist's perspective. Thus his or her related theory will lie within the parameters of such assumptions.

In nursing theories, some assumptions are usually made about the major concepts: Man, health, environment, and nursing. The human being is usually described as having certain general characteristics, which are applicable to both the client and the nurse. Assumptions about health—perhaps stated as wellness versus illness—are also usually made, and some theorists even describe the changed character of human beings when health is impaired. The environment may be labeled "society," "context," or "situation." The goals or roles of nursing are also a common topic for assumptions in nursing theories.

Theorists who have produced clear statements of assumption can provide us with good examples of what is involved in this process. For example, Newman makes the following assumptions about human beings and health:

1. Health encompasses conditions heretofore described as illness, or in medical terms, pathology.
2. These "pathological" conditions can be considered a manifestation of the total pattern of the individual.
3. The pattern of the individual that eventually manifests itself as pathology is primary and exists prior to structural or functional changes.
4. Removal of the pathology in itself will not change the pattern of the individual.
5. If becoming "ill" is the only way an individual's pattern can manifest itself, then that is health for that person.
6. Health is the expansion of consciousness.[11]

Parse states similar yet slightly different assumptions about Man, health, and environment for her nursing theory of Man-Living-Health.

1. Man is coexisting while coconstituting rhythmical patterns with the environment.
2. Man is an open being, freely choosing meaning in situation, bearing responsibility for decisions.
3. Man is a living unity continuously coconstituting patterns of relating.
4. Man is transcending multidimensionally with the possibles.
5. Health is an open process of becoming, experienced by Man.
6. Health is a rhythmically coconstituting process of the Man-environment interrelationship.
7. Health is Man's patterns of relating value priorities.
8. Health is an intersubjective process of transcending the possibles.
9. Health is unitary Man's negentropic unfolding.[12]

Travelbee makes the following assumptions about nursing:

The purpose of nursing is to assist an individual or family to present or cope with the experience of illness and suffering and, if necessary, to assist the individual or family to find meaning in these experiences. . . . the purpose of nursing is achieved through the establishment of a nurse-patient relationship.[13]

And Rogers states that·

The concern of nursing is with man in his entirety, his wholeness. Nursing's body of scientific knowledge seeks to describe, explain, and predict about human beings.[14]

Generally, then, as we read nursing theories, we can expect to find assumptions that relate to the central concerns of nursing, just as other disciplines focus theoretical assumptions on the central concerns that are unique to them.

LIMITATIONS OR EXCLUSIONS

In this chapter we are concerned only about assumptions that are associated with theories. Thus we can eliminate other definitions of the term, those whose meanings are considered outside the scope of our definition. For example, a person may "assume" a role, thus feigning a certain type of behavior. Or by "assuming" we can seize or usurp another's possession, place, or powers by force or without authorization. By another definition we "assume" responsibility or debts for another, taking them over as if they were our own. These meanings are all inappropriate to any discussion of assumptions in the realm of theories, and consequently we would eliminate them early in our consideration of theoretical assumptions.

Often it is difficult to distinguish a theorist's assumptions from his or her relationship statements or hypotheses; these differ in several ways. Relationship statements show changes in associations among major concepts of a theory. These are derived from assumptions regarding concepts and their relationships, and lead to hypotheses that predict future behavior or events regarding an interaction or movement among concepts. Relationship statements and hypotheses have to do with the internal functioning of a theory, not its basic assumptions. Thus assumptions tend to be statements that are static or factual in nature; they describe the way things are believed to be. In contrast, relationship statements and hypotheses tend to describe movement or change among concepts within the parameters established by assumptions. When trying to distinguish between them, sometimes the tense of the verb that is used can be a clue. Verbs that denote movement or change usually are found in relationship statements and hypotheses, whereas verbs that are associated with assumptions tend to be static and descriptive.

King provides a very clear example of the difficulties in distinguishing between assumptions, relationship statements, and hypotheses in her theory of goal attainment. In this theory, she makes the following statement as an assumption: "Perceptions of nurse and of client influence the interaction process."[15] Here the verb "influence" means that one thing is having an effect on another; it denotes some co-related change between two concepts. Thus we identify this statement not as an assumption but as a relationship statement. Generally, assumptions are statements about the way things are, about how things exist or can be perceived, not about how things relate to one another. Thus King's statement clearly demonstrates how easy it is to mistake a relationship statement for an assumption, or vice versa. A simple statement of assumption that probably captures King's intent is: "Nurses and clients can perceive one another with various degrees of accuracy."

A relationship statement that King derives from the assumption is that "if perceptual accuracy is present in nurse-client interactions, (then) transactions will occur."[16] Assumptions tend to be relatively simple statements of factual information, while relationship statements tend to follow predictable patterns. In the statement above, King has used the "If . . , then . . ." pattern. Other patterns for relationship statements are presented later in this text.

King's relationship statement can also be restated as a prediction. As such it becomes a hypothesis for research purposes: "Perceptual accuracy in nurse-patient interactions increases mutual goal setting."[17] As a prediction, this hypothesis can be tested in a research project to determine the degree to which the relationship statement is an accurate view of reality. This is the process of validating a theory. The assumptions, however, are not validated or tested.

While there may be other limitations or exclusions in the use of the term "assuming," the above discussion presents distinctions in meanings that we have found to be important in understanding theories and theory development in nursing.

ACCOMPLISHMENT, ROLE, AND FUNCTION

One purpose of assumptions is to set external and internal parameters for a theory.[18] This allows us to evaluate and criticize that theory. The degree to which assumptions seem to be consistent with our own experience of reality is indicative of external validity. For example, one of the external criticisms of some nursing theories is that the theorist describes what *should* or *must* be done by the nurse. The use of these terms is indicative of standards and expectations that may not exist or with which some may disagree. Theories that tend to be externally valid tend to describe what is or what *happens*, regardless of standards, expectations, or rules.

To evaluate a theory internally, we need to think about the assumptions it makes and decide whether or not the remainder of the theory seems to logically follow from them. For example, if it were assumed that we could go down to the Mississippi River and break off a chunk of water in July, then this implies that we would have chunky warm water for swimming, boating, fishing, and water skiing. If such were the case, we would need to perform all these activities very differently. We might even *chew* our morning coffee if we followed this assumption to its logical conclusion. Obviously, then, this is a ridiculous assumption. But from this example we can see that the degree to which we can accept the assumptions of a theory is an aid in our intuitive evaluation of the theory's validity, of its "goodness of fit" with reality.

Another function of assumptions is to guide and influence the research that will validate a particular theory.[19] In a sense, these assumptions limit the research, making it cover only the territory included in the assumptions. Fox suggests using the following five words to help identify covert assumptions and the limitations imposed by them: "who," "what," "where," "when," and "how."[20] Through assumptions, for example, a nursing theorist may limit a theory to situations in community health settings. From this it would logically follow that the researcher would need to select as subjects the clients and nurses from such settings. The assumptions also identify the kinds of data to collect and under what circumstances. Thus assumptions help guide and focus the research process so that only relevant activities are involved.

Still another role of assumptions is to aid in communicating clearly to professional colleagues and others the values and perspectives of the theorist. As Ackerman and Lohnes remind us, values can change with time, and for this reason we need to be explicit about how good or preferable something is.[21] In addition, Fox states that the soundest assumptions are based on previous research.[22] However, theories may also be based on the theorist's own experiences and observations.

Assumptions provide a trail of thinking for the reader to follow. Generally, it would seem that the degree to which the theorist can reveal through statements of assumptions the values, previous research, and experiences that have influenced the development of a theory to that degree the theory can be clearly communicated and understood by others.

ANALOGIES AND METAPHORS

Analogies and metaphors can be used to help us define assumptions. In Chapter 6, for example, we used the analogy of a theory being like a spotlight on a stage. To extend that analogy, we can think here of assumptions as being the stage itself. Assumptions limit the extent of a theory just as the floor and drapery or scenery of a stage limit the extent to which rays of light can penetrate the area.

Assumptions can also be likened to a particular toy. You may remember having played as a child with a little box with several small balls, usually metal BBs or buckshot. The top of the box consisted of clear glass so that you could see the motion of the balls as the box was tilted about. The objective was to maneuver all the balls into the holes in the bottom of the box. This entire toy can be considered to be like a theory: the sides and bottom of the box are analogous to assumptions; the little balls are analogous to concepts moving about within the parameters of the box. Remember that assumptions are descriptive statements that provide the framework within which concepts exist and interact. The framework does not move. Instead we focus on the phenomenon movement of the concepts. In the diagram in Figure 8, the solid line indicates the framework provided by the assumptions. The circles within the framework represent theoretical concepts, and the arrows indicate movement or some relationship between the concepts that is changing. These, then are examples of analogies that we can use in defining assumptions.

AUTHORITY QUOTES

We noted many quotations from authorities earlier in this chapter. These are statements that seem to provide succinct perspectives about assumptions in nursing and other disciplines.

SET OF ELEMENTS

While there may be sets of elements for the concept "assuming" proposed by authorities on theory development and analysis, in our search of the literature none were found. Thus we offer the following set of elements, which we believe will be helpful to the student of theories in understanding assumptions.

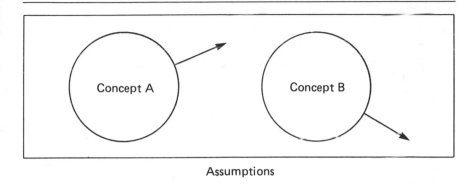

Assumptions

Figure 8. Assumptions analogy.

Observing. We first perceive some phenomenon, event, or occurrence in reality. Perceiving includes visually seeing, "here and now" experiencing, and a cognitive awareness of something. This can include all experiences, even extrasensory perception.

Remembering. We can also recall similar phenomena or events. We remember what is known from past experience or research, which may be relevant to our present experience.

Analoguing. We develop analogies about the present phenomenon and about similar phenomena. In the process, similarities and differences between them are identified and, through the use of metaphors, selected knowledge is brought to mind and given consideration in relation to this present phenomenon.

Expressing. Finally, a statement of presupposition is developed that is believed to be most reasonably true about the presently observed phenomenon. This statement represents the culmination of the assuming process—that is, it represents the expression of an assumption.

SUMMARY

In this chapter, we have presented a detailed analysis of the concept or element of a theory known as "assuming," defining it according to the nine ways of defining any concept. We have also proposed a set of four elements that describe the process of developing assumptions: observing, remembering, analoguing, and expressing. In the next chapter, we will deal in a similar manner with the second element of a theory, the concept.

NOTES

1. *Webster's New Collegiate Dictionary,* Henry Bosley Woolf, ed. (Springfield, Mass.: G. & C. Merriam, 1979), p. 68.
2. Abraham Kaplan, *The Conduct of Inquiry* (Scranton, Pa.: Chandler, 1964), p. 88.
3. Barbara J. Stevens, *Nursing Theory: Analysis, Application, Evaluation* (Boston: Little, Brown, 1979), p. 71.
4. Winona B. Ackerman and Paul R. Lohnes, *Research Methods for Nurses* (New York: McGraw-Hill, 1981), p. 15; David J. Fox, *Fundamentals of Research in Nursing,* 4th ed. (Norwalk, Conn.: Appleton-Century-Crofts, 1982), p. 44.
5. Kaplan, *Inquiry,* pp. 86–89.
6. Ibid., p. 87.
7. Abraham H. Maslow, *Motivation and Personality* (New York: Harper and Brothers, 1954).
8. William C. Schutz, *The Interpersonal Underworld* (Palo Alto, Calif.: Science and Behavior Books, 1966).
9. B. F. Skinner, *Science and Human Behavior* (New York: Macmillan, 1953).
10. Jean Piaget, *The Language and Thought of the Child* (New York: Harcourt, Brace, and World, 1926).
11. Margaret Newman, *Theory Development in Nursing* (Philadelphia: F. A. Davis, 1979), pp. 56–58.
12. Rosemarie Rizzo Parse, *Man-Living-Health: A Theory of Nursing* (New York: John Wiley, 1981), pp. 26–31.
13. Joyce Travelbee, *Interpersonal Aspects of Nursing* (Philadelphia: F. A. Davis, 1966), p. 13.
14. Martha E. Rogers, *An Introduction to the Theoretical Basis of Nursing* (Philadelphia: F. A. Davis, 1970), p. 3.
15. Imogene M. King, *A Theory for Nursing: Systems, Concepts, Processes* (New York: John Wiley, 1981), p. 143.
16. Ibid., p. 149.
17. Ibid., p. 156.
18. Stevens, *Nursing Theory,* pp. 20–21.
19. Ackerman and Lohnes, *Research Methods,* p. 17.
20. Fox, *Fundamentals of Research,* p. 44.
21. Ackerman and Lohnes, *Research Methods,* pp. 15–17.
22. Fox, *Fundamentals of Research,* pp. 116–117.

Concepts

8

The second sequential element in the process of developing a theory is conceptualizing. This involves attaching a term, word, or label to a thing, person, or event—in other words, classifying and describing a particular phenomenon. As in the case of assuming, we classify events, things, and people daily and seldom notice that we do so.

A large portion of our daily classifying and assigning tends to be evaluative in nature. For example, a neighbor recently asked her teen-aged daughter why she didn't accept an invitation to go out with a certain young man. The daughter responded indignantly, "With *that* turkey? That *geek?* Mother, really!" Thus the young man as a phe-nomenon was evaluated, classified, and labeled. The mother asked nothing more. She clearly did not want her daughter associating with turkeys and geeks; she classified these labels with terms more familiar to mothers, such as "creeps" and "weirdos" (obnoxious and unattrac-tive people). The assigning of labels to phenomena is not only helpful in mother-daughter communication; it is also a second essential ele-ment of theory development. Here, however, the evaluating takes on a somewhat different form as theorists evaluate the degree of congru-ency between reality and the concept rather than, say, degrees of attractiveness or "geekness" of potential dates. Thus in this chapter we will give careful attention to defining the conceptualizing process and to the term "concept," according to the nine ways of defining a concept.

DICTIONARY DEFINITIONS, SYNONYMS, AND DERIVATIONS

To conceptualize is to describe, classify, or designate. According to the dictionary definition, a concept is an abstract or generic idea or understanding, especially one that is derived from specific instances or occurrences. It is a thought or notion, an idea or conception.[1] The term "concept" is derived from the French word *conception*, which in turn is derived from the Latin *conceptio*, meaning to take to oneself. Among the synonyms for it are "idea," "thought," "notion," and "impression."[2]

Turning to the more specific definitions used in the scientific disciplines, we find similar terminology. Kaplan thinks of a concept as a family of conceptions. In his view, the act of conception belongs to a particular person, whereas a concept is an impersonal, timeless, "abstract construction" arising from those conceptions.[3] For example, each of us has conceptions of the black holes that have been discovered in outer space. As casual readers of science reports, most of us probably have some idea of what this phenomenon entails. But our layman's conception surely differs considerably from that of an astronomer or an astronaut. And the latter's conceptions are probably more consistent with the scientific definition of black holes than ours.

For scientific purposes, a concept is a timeless, abstract, impersonal theoretical term that serves as a norm and associates a label to specific phenomena. However, Reynolds states that it is the degree of agreement about a concept's nature and meaning that is the most important feature of scientific concepts. This is because scientists and theorists need to have some way of insuring that the scholarly speakers and receivers of scientific communications agree upon the meanings of the concepts they use.[4] Thus the careful defining of concepts assures the transmission of knowledge not only among contemporary scholars but also among past, present, and future scholars.

In the nursing literature, many authors often do not define the term "concept" specifically, nor do they clearly designate the concepts of a particular theory that is being presented.[5] This is in sharp contrast to King and Newman, who clearly identify the concepts that make up their respective theories.[6] In fact, Newman defines the term "concept" in the same way that Kerlinger does, as "an abstraction formed by generalization from particulars."[7]

It appears that at least one author in the nursing field has erred by describing the term "concept" as being a principle (a relationship statement) and a premise (an assumption).[8] Watson states that a concept is a "mental picture or a mental image, a word that symbolizes ideas and meanings and expresses an abstraction."[9] But Ackerman and Lohnes reject the term "concept" and use "construct" instead because they have found definitions of concepts insufficiently discriminatory.[10] For Diers, a concept is "simply a word to which meaning has been attached through formal definition or common usage . . . an abstraction, not directly observable," and a construct is "just a fancier kind of concept, one which has in it several concepts."[11]

Generally, it appears that in the discipline and profession of nursing scholars have not yet agreed upon the usage and definition of "concept" as a theoretical element. Therefore, for the purposes of clarity, we propose the following definition:

A concept is a term or word used to describe, classify, or designate a specific set of phenomena or a set of conceptions. It is a timeless, abstract, impersonal idea that serves as a norm. A set of concepts provides the necessary elements of theories and may have definitions unique and specific to particular theories. Theoretical concepts are relabeled "variables" when they are operationalized for research purposes.

This is not a unique definition. It is merely a restatement of traditional definitions of concepts found in dictionaries and other texts. In presenting it, we are reminded of critic Kenneth Burke's statement in reference to Aristotle's definition of tragedy: "A definition so sums things up that all properties attributed to the thing defined can be as though 'derived' from the definition."[12]

We propose that nursing as a discipline will be best served by the general acceptance of the traditional terminology used in theory development and research in the social and biological sciences—a position that is consistent with the eristic style of thinking. Thus, rather than developing a new system of terminology as suggested by Ackerman and Lohnes,[13] we suggest that greater attention be given to developing definitions of concepts that, as Burke suggests, sum things up. If our definitions are complete, then they will be sufficiently discriminatory to meet our theoretical and scientific needs. After all, Torres reminds us that the word "concept" has been used in nursing "for over fifty years without its having a specific meaning and will probably continue to do so for several more decades."[14]

OPERATIONAL DEFINITION

How a concept is operationally defined is of paramount importance in theory development and testing because in this process the researcher makes a "leap of faith" between the theoretical definition and the phenomenon with which the concept is to be associated. In order to make a concept "happen," we assign explicit meaning to that concept. Thus a set of instructions or operations needs to be clearly stated so that others within a discipline, particularly theorists and researchers, are able to replicate the phenomenon. This involves much more than simply using other words to define a word; rather, it involves specifying those activities, procedures, or operations that are necessary in order for us to observe the phenomenon for ourselves, to personally witness the concept happening. This linking between the theoretical concept and the operations from which observable data arise is referred to by some authors as the "rules of correspondence" or the "rules of interpretation."

There seem to be four elements to operational definitions: experimental, measuremental, administrative, and evaluative. Each of these elements will be discussed and related to nursing in the paragraphs that follow.[15]

Experimental

An experimental operational definition provides specific details or operations that are necessary for a concept to be manipulated or treated in some way so that it changes or varies. This represents the core of the theory-validating process. In the view of many scholars, the quality of research results rests upon the methods used to operationalize a theoretical concept under experimentally controlled conditions. Generally, research findings cannot rise above the validity of methodology.[16] Thus we need to be sure that our experiment is testing and measuring what we intend to test and measure; this is what "validity" means.[17]

Measuremental

A measuremental operational definition provides information about how a concept or variable can be measured. A variable is something that changes or varies, so in research a theoretical concept is often referred to by this term. A theoretical concept as a variable has values assigned to it so that the degree of change can be noted.

There are several ways in which we can think about a variable being measured. A *dichotomous variable* such as x has only two values, 1 and 2. For example, the variable "gender" can be either male or female.

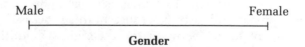

Similarly, the variable "employment" may be assigned either a "yes" or a "no" value.

A *polytomous variable* can have several values assigned to it. For example, a nurse may have graduated from a diploma program, an associate degree program, a generic baccalaureate program, or a "second step" baccalaureate program for RNs.

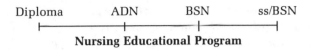

Nursing Educational Program

However, most variables can be theoretically considered as *continuous variables*. For example, intelligence has been conceptualized as a continuous variable with numerical gradations in value that are assigned in this fashion:

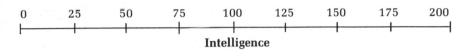

Intelligence

Values on a continuous variable may also be reassigned so that we have fewer categories to meet our research purposes:

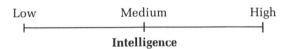

Intelligence

In this way, continuous variables may also be treated as dichotomous variables. However, the reverse is not also the case: a true dichotomous variable cannot become a continuous variable:

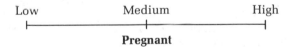

Pregnant

A woman is either pregnant or not; she cannot be a little bit pregnant.

According to Kerlinger, there are four categories of measurement: nominal, ordinal, interval, and ratio.[18] *Nominal* measurement is the lowest level of assigning value; it merely involves giving labels to categories. Thus members of a set are assigned letters of the alphabet, numbers, or names, permitting us to assign individual observations to a category. For example, people serving as subjects in a research project may be assigned subject numbers. In a similar fashion, patients in a hospital are assigned labels according to religious preference, degree of illness, and room number, and thus are nominally measured so that they can be counted and compared. Statistical tools often used at this level of measurement include percentage distributions, chi-square, and correlation coefficients.

Ordinal measurement involves rank ordering according to some property or characteristic of the set of objects. There are three ways in which this kind of measurement is usually done. We can determine that one object is greater than the next: $a > b, b > c, c > d$, and so on. We may also use a combination of two or more characteristics so that we get a combined value. For example, we can average state board examination scores to obtain one composite score to use in ranking a group of graduates. Or we can develop additional criteria, such as "less than" ($<$), "precedes," "is above" or "is superior to," or "is greater than" ($>$).

In using ordinal measurement, we must be very careful not to assume that the intervals between the values are equal. Remember, the rank-ordered scale doesn't have a zero point, so we don't know whether or not there are members of the set that have none, 0.0 or zero, of the characteristic that's being ordinally measured. Statistical tools often applied at this level of measurement include percentage distributions, correlational coefficients, and analysis of variance. However, the true magnitude of properties or characteristics is not established.

Interval measurement not only labels and rank orders but also provides equal distance between values on the scale of measurement. For example, thermometers measure a client's fever in terms of equal interval numbers, which can be added and subtracted. However, the units and zero points are arbitrarily established. Many more statistical tools can be used on concepts that are sufficiently defined to allow this level of measurement, but only an approximate statement can be made about the true value of the concept. This is about the best measurement scale available for most scientific work, but achieving this level of measurement is still rare in such fields as psychology, sociology, and most of the humanistic and social disciplines.

Ratio measurement is the highest level of measurement. The added feature here is that the absolute or natural zero is added, in addition to all of the characteristics of the lower-level measurement described above: equality in properties, rank order, equality of intervals, and equality of ratios. The absolute zero means that the researcher can provide for some object in the set having none of the property that's being measured. Thus the arithmetic operations of multiplication and division become possible. Furthermore, ratio measurement is distinctive in that the numerical values on the scale of measurement indicate actual amounts of the characteristic or quality being measured. Examples of such types of measurement include those determining length and width. Such precision is rare in the humanities and the social sciences.

Generally, it is true that the higher the level of measurement achieved, the greater the degree of representativeness of data according to numerical values. Thus as a more specific and accurate quality of data is required, ultimately a more precise research and/or theoretical statement becomes possible. However, absolute true measurement is considered beyond human achievement because of inevitable errors in measurement and fluctuations in data. Statistical theories and operations allow for this random error so that we achieve the best scientific statements we can.

Administrative

The administrative or management operational definition of a concept, according to Emmert and Brooks, consists of all the little details necessary to obtain the data.[19] For example, in nursing we must obtain numerous permissions from groups (such as the committee to protect human and animal subjects) and individuals (such as the heads of clinical services). This often involves considerable time and effort spent in corresponding, telephoning, and perhaps even defending a project before a committee. We must obtain consent from each subject and gain his or her cooperation in the research project. And we need to provide equipment and supplies that are appropriate for data collection. Then we need to code the data itself and prepare it for computer analysis. If we're fortunate enough to be funded by a grant, then careful fiscal accountability is also involved in the administrative operationalizing of a concept.

Evaluative

The evaluative operational definition involves setting up criteria for operationalizing a concept and devising some means whereby we can determine the degree to which the criteria are met. The criteria cited by Emmert and Brooks are those of Feigle, which were later modified by Bachrach.[20] These general criteria include the following characteristics for operational definitions: (1) logically consistent operations; (2) quantitative; (3) observable; (4) manipulatable experimentally; (5) intersubjective and repeatable; and (6) contributing to the development of laws or predictiveness. These general criteria are relatively easily achieved when dealing with observable data, as in the physical sciences and some areas of the behavioral sciences.

However, in nursing, phenomena and concepts need to be perceived as existing on a continuum of abstraction.

Empirically observable	Indirectly observable	Theoretically observable
Concrete	Sign	Abstract
Artifact	Instrumentation	Symbolic
Objective		Subjective

Some of the concepts in nursing are concrete and observable, as in the measurement of decubitus ulcers. Others are indirectly observable through signs and instrumentation, as in using fetal heart monitors. But there is also a need to recognize and explore phenomena that are very abstract and subjective, as well as unique to nursing. The Nursing Development Conference Group, chaired by Orem, represents a current effort by nurse scholars to identify concepts that are relevant to nursing and of significant importance to the development of theoretical perspectives for research and practice.[21] It seems highly probable that unique, abstract, and subjective concepts will be identified in nursing, concepts that have either not been operationalized by other disciplines or that have been operationalized in ways that are not applicable to nursing. Thus there is a need for nurses to develop criteria specifically applicable to nursing concept operationalization.

One example of such a concept is that of anger. Although anger is a common feeling expressed frequently by most of us, a review of the literature failed to produce a means of operationalizing anger experimentally to determine the effects of its expression by peers and colleagues upon people generally or upon nurses specifically.[22] No criterion had been accepted as adequate to define the phenomenon being measured: everyday, garden-variety anger—just foot-stamping, teeth-gritting, fist-clenching, red-faced, door-slamming, hissie-fit "mad." These kinds of criteria are acceptable in everyday life but not in research. This is a human feeling assumed to be reflected and expressed in the test situation according to the theory. For research to support a theory, however, the scientific scholar needs some measurable indicators or signs that the concept is "happening" in the test situation.

Drawing from discussions of construct validation by Cronbach and Meehl, who define a construct as "some postulated attribute of people assumed to be reflected in test performance,"[23] nurse researcher Duldt identified questions or criteria that seemed appropriate for validating the concept of anger. Would trained judges be able to identify written messages as non-anger, maintenance mode anger, and destructive mode anger? Would subjects be able to identify the messages as expressions of anger? Would the subjects be able to distinguish between the two modes of anger in such a manner that it would be reflected in task performance, ratings, and other responses? And since the subjects were to respond to the written messages, another test would be whether or not the trained judges would be able to classify the subjects' written messages according to the various modes of anger expressions that Duldt had theoretically defined. The answers to these questions were determined by having many groups of judges, trained and untrained, categorize experimental messages until almost total agreement could be obtained among the judges. This process is called Q-sorting. The intensity of anger communicated was also determined by a series of Q-sorting and ratings by still other judges. Finally, the classification of the subjects' written messages was achieved by trained judges who attained an inter-rater reliability of .90 and higher. An analysis of the subjects' various responses yielded covert evidence of desired differences between the various experimental messages. Having verified the theoretical concept of anger in this manner, other research questions were identified and more studies were conducted until a theory of anger was developed, a new concept—that of anger dismay—was identified, and considerable information was accumulated about anger in nursing practice.[24]

This is an example of a very abstract concept about human feelings or pathos and its expression or logos being validated by judges who identify a particular phenomenon and agree that it does in fact go with a particular concept or word. Q-sorting is only one technique of achieving this. Semantic differentials also identify and measure the meaning of words through the use of multiple bipolar adjectives. And attitude and rating scales can be applied to Likert scales.[25]

Some important yet very abstract and subjective concepts—such as comfort, authenticity, caring, touching, acceptance, and positive regard—still need to be explored by nurse scholars. But they will need to be very attentive in developing criteria for evaluating these operational definitions for nursing research purposes.

A Recap of Operational Definitions

In summary, all four aspects of operationally defining a concept—experimental, measuremental, administrative, and evaluative—are of paramount importance in theoretical statements and in research efforts to support such statements. This linking between theoretical concepts and research (and practice) operations lies at the heart of the development of a sound knowledge base for any discipline. If such a "leap of faith" between the concept and the test event fails, the ensuing research efforts will be of little value.

In using the eristic model of thinking in such disciplines as speech communication, social psychology, and sociology, the preferred research strategy is to identify one concept and determine how changing amounts of this concept influence only one or two other concepts.[26] It is proposed that this approach is particularly applicable to the discipline and profession of nursing.

SCOPE AND LIMITATIONS

In developing a concept, a set of utterances is grouped together and identified as a term or word. This word or concept is then applied, often arbitrarily, to a phenomenon. A concept, according to Kaplan, is an impersonal, timeless norm.[27] There is usually a naturalness about a concept in that attributes used as a basis of classification or as elements of one concept are often related to attributes that are conceptualized elsewhere in our thinking. In other words, things are grouped together because they seem to resemble one another.[28] As suggested in Chapter 3, we can compare the scope of a concept to the drawing of a circle, thoughtfully placing all the aspects and meanings we intend to convey within that circle. By the same token, we can limit or exclude those aspects and meanings of a phenomenon and concept that we do not wish to convey by placing them outside the circle.

Using the scope and limitations of anger as an example of this process, we can see that such activity can readily become problematic. After all, researchers may view the same phenomena, but they may conceptualize from differing perspectives. Duldt provides this example:

If one were to consider anger on a continuum from zero to ten, there are a number of concepts which could be related to anger in a curvilinear fashion. The assertion of leadership, for example, might be viewed as requiring some degree of arousal similar to anger, perhaps about three on the scale. If expressions of assertiveness are sufficiently credible, others can be persuaded, motivated, or, as Schachter et al.[29] state, induced to greater productivity. Expressions of anger, especially by a high status member, can be persuasive and induce conformity to norms. This might occur at about five on the scale. All of these concepts are more or less constructive. At some point, however, perhaps around eight, expression of anger may become too strong so that credibility is lost. It may become abrasive, offensive, and destructive to group processes. In short, while some researchers may label the phenomenon they are observing as low-level anger, hostility, antagonism, aggression, and rage, they may in fact be observing what others may be labeling leadership, persuasion, motivation, and conviction. This seems particularly true of studies in which attitude tests, rating scales, and other subjective measurement methods are used.[30]

Thus the differing perspectives of researchers can lead to an overlapping of definitions, making it difficult to know what individual theorists and researchers are including and excluding in the scope of their conceptual and even operational definitions.

In nursing, similar problems are evident. Just as clinical psychologists and physicians have been known to disagree about whether specific problems, such as sexual impotency, are psychological or medical in nature, so nurses have had difficulty defending their positions on what is to be included in nursing and what belongs to other professional practice disciplines. Indeed, nurses disagree among themselves about the conceptual territory of nursing versus non-nursing. For example, Johnson states that historically, nursing has not been a highly valued service by society, that it has not been viewed as critical in comparison with other practice disciplines such as medicine. Rather, it has been viewed as a very practical rather than intellectual service, and consequently its development as a discipline with a strong knowledge base has not been supported. More important, however, as Johnson points out, is the fact that the services provided by nursing involve such a wide scope of phenomena of an abstract nature that it has been particularly difficult to determine the scope and limitations of the field. Furthermore, as Johnson states, there are no "scientific giants in nursing's heritage on whose shoulders present-day investigators can stand."[31]

However, there does seem to be some agreement in nursing on what the focus of the discipline and profession is to be—on the *person who is ill,* on the client. And there seems to be general agreement that the major concepts of theoretical concern included in the nursing paradigm are the human being or Man, the nurse, the environment or society, and health. A paradigm establishes the phenomenon or concepts to be considered within the boundaries of a discipline. It gives direction about the methodologies and processes used within the discipline or profession. Generally, nursing is focused on the analysis of interactions between and among these four concepts.[32] (See Figure 9.) "Models" of theories provide one general classification of individual theories. A model provides a relational approach for a paradigm.[33] Relational approaches include, among other things, a developmental perspective of phenomena, a mechanistic view, or a systems view. While providing some relational characteristics of specific theories, the primary role and function of models is to guide theory development; such models are usually used in all academic disciplines. (See Figure 9.)

"Conceptual frameworks" are often noted in the nursing literature. In these frameworks, concepts are defined and explored to identify conditions and factors that are necessary to change or influence the concept. While linkages may be identified between one concept and one or more others, theoretical statements of relationships have not yet been made; thus the criteria of a theory are not met. However, with the conceptual framework as a focal point, scholars may be able to develop definitions and linkages among concepts to develop a theory that can be tested. Conceptual frameworks are often used by a group such as a faculty as a basis for developing nursing curricula, particularly if the faculty does not wish to be committed to one nursing theory. Rather, they choose concepts of particular relevance to nursing, as noted above. Similarly, a nursing staff may develop a conceptual framework for providing nursing care within a health agency. By this means, they are able to refer to the theories of their choice, which use these concepts or synonyms thereof, in organizing course content and curriculum design. This seems to be another sign that nursing as a discipline is at the preconceptual level of development. The reports of the Nursing Theories Conference Group and the Nursing Development Conference Group seem to document all too well the ongoing struggle to determine the scope and limitations of fundamental concepts in nursing.[34]

ACCOMPLISHMENT, ROLE, AND FUNCTION

The role and function of a concept in theory development is to label phenomena. Thus concepts function to "mark paths by which we may freely move into logical space."[35] Meanings are assigned to concepts, yet the meaning remains in people rather than in the words. Judgments are made and actions are taken based on the meanings that are assigned to concepts. In other words, meanings vary with the context.

The range of possible functions of a concept can be very broad and is related to the perceptual cues that are received from various phenomena. For the scientist this scope can be much more selective than it is for others. Concepts provide a prescription for organizing and ordering our experiences in day-to-day living. In addition, concepts categorize and classify information and subjects to serve whatever purposes we intend. As timeless and impersonal norms, concepts are linguistic instruments of science to which meanings are assigned and validated through testing.[36]

ANALOGIES AND METAPHORS

A number of analogies and metaphors have been used in the discussions above. For example, we have referred to concepts as instru-

Characteristic	Paradigm	Model	Conceptual Framework	Theory
Guide for nature, goals, methodology	Yes	No	No	No
Assumptions	Maybe	Yes	Yes	Yes
Defines concepts	Yes	Yes	Yes	Yes
Relationship statements	No	Yes	Yes	Yes
Testable and refutable	No	No	No	Yes
Establishes boundary of discipline/profession	Yes	No	No	No
Contributes to knowledge base	No	No	No	Yes
Guide for theory development	Yes	Yes	No	No
Guide for practice	Maybe	Maybe	No	Probably
Guide for program or service	Maybe	Maybe	Yes	Maybe
Ownership	Members of a discipline or a profession	All academic investigators	Small group i.e., faculty or nursing service	Individual theorist

Figure 9. *Differentiation of characteristics of paradigm, model, conceptual framework, and theory.*

ments. In addition, conceptualizing has been likened to building a fence around a phenomenon to distinguish what is to be included and what excluded. Concepts can also be thought of as the building blocks of theories. Generally, there seem to be very few analogies and metaphors about concepts in the literature, particularly the nursing literature. Like other linguistic tools, we tend to use concepts regularly, but we tend not to think about them very often.

AUTHORITY QUOTES

In the paragraphs above, we have already presented numerous quotations by authorities. Additional statements of significance include the following by Kerlinger:

The scientist . . . realizes that the concepts he is using are man-made terms that may or may not exhibit a close relation to reality.

A concept expresses an abstraction formed by generalization from particulars. . . . A construct is a concept. It has the added meaning, however, of having been deliberately and consciously invented or adopted for a specific scientific purpose.[37]

A notable quotation by Emmert and Brooks declares that:

Operational definitions (sometimes called "epistemic" definitions) serve as a bridge between theoretically defined constructs possessing constitutive meaning and observable data. Sometimes operational definitions are called "rules of correspondence" or "rules of interpretation" because they define, or at least partially define, certain theoretical constructs by connecting or linking them to observable data or operations.[38]

Thayer takes a more personal perspective:

The only reality upon which an individual can base his behavior is his own reality—*his* conceptual structuring of the world, *his* model or image of it, *his* expectations about the future.[39]

Again, we would caution you to note the degree of credibility attributed to an authority in evaluating the worth of his or her quotation.

SET OF ELEMENTS

While there may be sets of elements that describe the process of developing a concept, we found none in our search of the literature. Thus we propose the following process set of six elements as a sequential way of thinking about concept formulation: experiencing, comparing, labeling, norming, communicating, and refining.

Experiencing. In this step, something happens. A phenomenon is sensed in some way. The experience is often shared by two or more individuals.

Comparing. Having shared the experience, one individual, a theorist and researcher, turns to the colleague and asks, "Did you see what I saw?" In the ensuing dialogue, comparisons are made of perceptions about the experience.

Labeling. In the dialogue, a symbol or sign—a concept—is selected to signify this and all similar experiences.

Norming. One result of comparing and labeling perceptions is the development of a consensus of opinions about the facts and meaning or implications of the experience.

Communicating. These individuals and others henceforth are able to talk about the experience as abstracted by the symbols, label, or concept. Comparisons, impressions, characteristics and other aspects of the experienced phenomenon might be shared, thus expanding knowledge.

Refining. Once established, the defining of the concept can be refined. Quantification of the concept at the nominal, ordinal, interval, or ratio levels may be determined,[40] and the scope and limitations of the concept may become more discretely demarcated.

This total process of concept formulation ultimately establishes a relationship between the concept and the phenomena that are experienced, resulting in a comprehensive definition of the concept.

SUMMARY

In this chapter, we have presented an extensive discussion of the second major element of a theory, the concept. We have defined it according to the nine ways of defining any concept, and we have made a number of statements regarding the degree to which concept formulization has occurred in nursing as a discipline and profession. We have also proposed a set of six elements that describe the concept formulization process. In the chapter that follows, we will discuss in a similar manner the third element of a theory, the relationship statement.

NOTES

1. *Webster's New Collegiate Dictionary,* Henry Bosley Woolf, ed. (Springfield, Mass.: G. & C. Merriam, 1979), p. 231.
2. Ibid.; *Webster's New Dictionary of Synonyms,* Phillip B. Grove, ed. (Springfield, Mass.: G. & C. Merriam, 1968), p. 171.
3. Abraham Kaplan, *The Conduct of Inquiry* (Scranton, Pa: Chandler, 1964), p. 49.
4. Paul Davidson Reynolds, *A Primer in Theory Construction* (Indianapolis: Bobbs-Merrill, 1971), pp. 46–48.
5. Dorothea E. Orem, *Nursing: Concepts of Practice* (New York: McGraw-Hill, 1971); Josephine G. Patterson and Loretta Zderad, *Humanistic Nursing* (New York: John Wiley, 1976); Joyce Travelbee, *Interpersonal Aspects of Nursing* (Philadelphia: F. A. Davis, 1966).
6. Imogene M. King, *A Theory for Nursing: Systems, Concepts, Process* (New York: John Wiley, 1981), pp. 144–149; Margaret Newman, *Theory Development in Nursing* (Philadelphia: F. A. Davis, 1979), p. 59.
7. Ibid., p. 7; Fred N. Kerlinger, *Foundations of Behavioral Research* (New York: Holt, Rinehart and Winston, 1973), p. 28.

8. Barbara J. Stevens, *Nursing Theory: Analysis, Application, Evaluation* (Boston: Little, Brown, 1979), p. 32.

9. Jean Watson, *Nursing: The Philosophy and Science of Caring* (Boston: Little, Brown, 1979), pp. 61–62.

10. Winona B. Ackerman and Paul R. Lohnes, *Research Methods for Nurses* (New York: McGraw-Hill, 1981) pp. 11–12.

11. Donna Diers, *Research in Nursing* (Philadelphia: J. B. Lippincott, 1979), p. 69.

12. Kenneth Burke, *Language as Symbolic Action* (Berkeley: University of California Press, 1968), p. 3.

13. Ackerman and Lohnes, *Research Methods*, pp. 11–12.

14. Gertrude Torres, "The Place of Concepts and Theories Within Nursing," in Julia B. George, chairperson, Nursing Theories Conference Group, *Nursing Theories: The Base for Professional Nursing Practice* (Englewood Cliffs, N.J.: Prentice-Hall, 1980), p. 2.

15. The authors have been strongly influenced by Emmert and Brooks and by Kerlinger. We credit their work for most of the distinctions made in this section. The specific works consulted include: Phillip Emmert and William D. Brooks, *Methods of Research in Communication* (Boston: Houghton Mifflin, 1970), pp. 30–41; and Kerlinger, *Foundations of Behavioral Research*, pp. 28–46.

16. Emmert and Brooks, *Methods of Research in Communication*, p. 31.

17. Kerlinger, *Foundations of Behavioral Research*, p. 457.

18. Ibid., pp. 434–438.

19. Emmert and Brooks, *Methods of Research in Communication*, p. 36.

20. Ibid., p. 34; H. Feigl, "Operationism and the Scientific Method," *Psychological Review* 52 (1945):250–259; A. J. Bachrach, *Psychological Research* (New York: Random House, 1965), p. 82.

21. Dorothea E. Orem, ed., *Concept Formulization in Nursing: Process and Product*, 2nd ed. (Boston: Little, Brown, 1979).

22. Bonnie Weaver Grant (Duldt), "Anger, Cohesiveness, and Productivity in Small Task Groups" (Unpublished doctoral dissertation, University of Kansas, Lawrence, 1977) in *Dissertation Abstracts International* (University Microfilms International No. 7824799, 39, 3916A, January 1979).

23. Lee J. Cronback and Paul E. Meehl, "Construct Validity in Psychological Tests," *Psychological Bulletin* 52 (4): 283–284.

24. Bonnie W. Duldt, "Anger: An Occupational Hazard for Nurses," *Nursing Outlook* 29, no. 9 (September 1981):510–518; Bonnie W. Duldt, "Anger: An Alienating Communication Hazard for Nurses," *Nursing Outlook* 29, no. 11 (November 1981):640–644; "Commentary," *Nursing Outlook* 30, no. 2 (February 1982):84–85; Bonnie Weaver Duldt, "Helping Nurses to Cope with the Anger-Dismay Syndrome," *Nursing Outlook* 30, no. 3 (March 1982):168–174.

25. Emmert and Brooks, *Methods of Research in Communication*, pp. 165–180, 181–196, and 197–213.

26. Leonard C. Hawes, *Pragmatics of Analoguing: Theory and Model Con-

struction in Communication (Reading, Mass.: Addison-Wesley, 1975), p. 11.

27. Kaplan, *Conduct of Inquiry*, p. 49.
28. Ibid., p. 50.
29. Stanley Schachter, Norris Ellerton, Dorothy McBride, and Doris Gregory, "An Experimental Study of Cohesiveness and Productivity," *Human Relations* 4 (1951):229–238.
30. Grant (Duldt), "Anger, Cohesiveness, and Productivity in Small Task Groups," p. 7.
31. Dorothy E. Johnson, "Development of Theory: A Requisite for Nursing as a Primary Health Profession," *Nursing Research* 23 (September-October 1974):208–209.
32. Janice A. Thibodeau. *Nursing Models: Analysis and Evaluation* (Monterey, Calif.: Wadsworth Health Sciences Division, 1983), pp. 2–14.
33. Ibid., p. 9.
34. George, *Nursing Theories*; Orem, *Concept Formulization in Nursing*.
35. Kaplan, *Conduct of Inquiry*, p. 52.
36. Ibid., pp. 46–52.
37. Kerlinger, *Foundations of Behavioral Research*, pp. 3, 28–29.
38. Emmert and Brooks, *Methods of Research in Communication*, p. 34.
39. Lee Thayer, *Communication and Communication Systems* (Homewood, Ill.: Richard D. Irwin, 1968), p. 45.
40. Reynolds, *A Primer in Theory Construction*, pp. 57–64.

Relationship Statements 9

The third sequential element in the process of formulating a theory is developing relationship statements between two or more concepts. Just as assumptions provide the perspective or framework for a theory, and just as operationalizing concepts provide the core of theory validation, so relationships provide a theory with meaning.

As in the cases of assuming and of classifying phenomena into conceptual categories, so too do we relate things in our daily lives. For example, before asking an attractive young lady out to dinner, a young man usually looks in his billfold to see whether or not he has enough money to pay for both dinners. If he has enough, then he can invite her; if he doesn't, then he can't. Only an "air head" gets things like this mixed up. People learn rather early in life that it's important to check out relevant facts before taking action. While shopping, a young woman is a real "space cadet" if she doesn't check the size and price of a blouse before she takes it to the cash register to pay for it. In fact, we expect people to relate things, to keep their act together, to pay attention to what's going on. And in professional practice of any nature, we also expect the practitioner to be exceptionally capable of relating important facts and of knowing the implications arising from their relationship. A nurse is really "spacey" if he or she doesn't listen for bowel sounds in the postoperative patient's abdomen before removing the levine tube. Theorists provide us with formal statements of relationships among important concepts and help us understand the meanings and implications of those concepts. This in turn may provide some predictability for the outcome of action or inaction on our part in professional practice contexts.

In this chapter, we will define what a theoretical relationship statement is according to the nine ways of defining any concept. We will also give guidelines for identifying the various forms that are used in making statements of relationship. This will also provide an awareness of the close ties between theory development and research.

DICTIONARY DEFINITIONS, SYNONYMS, AND DERIVATIONS

According to the dictionary, a relationship refers to a logical or natural association between two or more things. It indicates that one has relevance to another, that there is a connection. In other words, there is some aspect, characteristic, or quality that connects two or more things as belonging or working together, as in the relationship between time and space.[1] A statement, of course, is the act of presenting a report in written or oral form.[2] Thus a relationship statement, for our purposes here, is a written or oral report of an association between two or more concepts within the framework of a specific set of theoretical assumptions.

The term "relate" is derived from the Latin *relatus*, meaning to carry back.[3] Apparently the word refers to carrying back messages, telling stories, or giving an account of an event. The synonyms for it are numerous because the Latin is also applicable to family ties through marriage, to interpersonal communication (relationships) between people, and even to affiliations developed between individuals or groups. Some of the synonyms that are germane to theoretical relationship statements include "associate," "link," "connect," "join," "conjoin," "combine," "unite," and "correspond."[4]

In the disciplines that are related to nursing, a more pertinent definition of theoretical relationship is found in Kaplan's discussions of measurement.[5] Here we need to assume that the way in which we have defined theoretical concepts and the knowledge we have accumulated about the concepts will enable us to measure them. In this context, measurement is viewed as the assignment of numbers to aspects of the concepts according to a rule of magnitude. The rule of assignment allows "one to one correspondence," meaning that only one object or aspect of a concept may be mapped into any one point. The numbers, then, "map into abstract space" the structure of relationships among concepts; thus, "counting and measuring are regarded as the necessary conditions for scientific progress."[6]

Measurement allows for standardization, for more precise descriptions, and, ultimately, for the statement of principles or laws.[7] Theoretical relationship statements therefore are patterned after the relationships among numbers. For this reason it becomes important for the student of theories to be aware of numerical relationships in order to more easily identify and recognize the patterns of the relationship statements used by theorists.

In a review of the nursing literature, theoretical relationship statements are not defined as a rule. One exception, however, is the defining of hypotheses, which are theoretical relationship statements rephrased into specific measurable and testable statements of expected outcomes for testing in specific research projects. Ackerman and Lohnes discuss hypotheses rather extensively,[8] and Diers distinguishes a first level of research, (asking "What *is* this?") from a second level (asking "What is *happening?*"). Thus the distinction is made between descriptive research and research designed to identify relationships between concepts.[9] Roy and Newman are two nursing authors who specifically associate theoretical statements of relationships with patterns of relationships in statistics or logic.[10] The knowledge and understanding of the association between statements relating concepts and patterns of relationship among numbers is of paramount importance in understanding the operationalization of relationship statements.

OPERATIONAL DEFINITION

While many things can be related, our focus here is the relationship between two or more concepts. Theoretical statements of these relationships take rather classic forms having relevance to statistical operations. In the following paragraphs, we will present a brief description of those forms that are frequently seen in many modern theories. For our discussions, we shall use the letters X, Y, and Z to represent three separate concepts of a theory.

The first form concerns whether or not the concepts occur. Hawes divides these logical terms into three categories:[11]

1. Either X or Y exists (the disjunctive form).
2. Both X and Y occur together (the conjunctive form).
3. If X occurs, then Y occurs (the conditional or causal form).

A relationship is in the *disjunctive* form if, for example, a window is either open (X) or closed (Y), or if a woman is either pregnant (X) or not pregnant (Y). In other words, concept X cannot occur if concept Y is present. In the *conjunctive* form, an example of a relationship statement might be: when I have a broken leg (X), I am unable to walk (Y). Thus when concept X occurs, we can expect concept Y also to occur. In the *conditional* or *causal* form, a relationship between stress and adaptation might be stated as follows: if stress (X) occurs, then adaptation (Y) will occur. In other words, when X occurs, its very presence will cause Y to happen. These forms generally represent a simple relationship between concepts and do not provide for levels, gradations, or varying amounts of each concept. This is provided in the next kind of form.

The second kind is the *correlational* or *association* form, as described by Paul Reynolds.[12] It shows variations in the amounts of each concept in relation to one another:

1. Positive or direct: $(\uparrow X, \uparrow Y)$, $(\sim X, \sim Y)$, or $(\downarrow X, \downarrow Y)$.
2. Inverse: $(\uparrow X, \downarrow Y)$ or $(\downarrow X, \uparrow Y)$.

The *positive* or *direct correlation* means that both X and Y occur in high amounts, low amounts, or are unchanged ($\sim$) in the presence of each other. The *inverse correlation* means that X occurs in high amounts while Y occurs in low amounts or vice versa. The statistical tool or analysis for this form is the Pearson Product-Moment correlation and similar procedures.

Wike states that the correlation form provides information about two aspects of the relationship, direction and strength.[13] Thus the Pearson Product-Moment Correlation Coefficient, often indicated by the letter "r," has an index that ranges from a positive to a negative one:

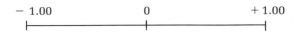

$$-1.00 \qquad\qquad 0 \qquad\qquad +1.00$$

An "r" of +1.00 is a perfect direct relationship, 0 indicates no relationship, and −1.00 is a perfect inverse relationship. The sign indicates the direction of the relationship and the numerical value indicates the strength. Generally the correlational or associational form is an important type of relationship pattern that is commonly used in theoretical statements of relationship. Other forms which build on this one and become more complex, are the deterministic and the probabilistic forms.

A *deterministic* statement limits the scope within which the relationship can occur. It is analogous to the reservation in the development of an argument as discussed in Chapter 4, and can be expressed in the following way: under conditions $(C_1, \ldots, C_n)$, if concept X occurs, then concept Y will occur. That is, under $C_1, \ldots, C_n$, if X, then Y. An example of this form would be: under conditions of good health (C_1), adequate diet (C_2), and reasonable amounts of rest (C_3) and exercise (C_4), if severe stress (X) occurs, then adaptation (Y) in the normal human being will readily occur in proportion (that is, under $C_1, \ldots, C_4$, if X, then Y). While the deterministic statement provides considerable information about relationships between concepts, another statement provides even more.

The *probabilistic* statement predicts the degree of truth of the relationship between the concepts. This statement builds on the deterministic statement and is analogous to the qualifier in the development of an argument in eristic thinking as discussed in Chapter 4. A probabilistic statement states that under certain conditions $(C_1, \ldots, C_n)$, if concept X occurs, then concept Y will occur with a certain degree of probability (P). That is, under $C_1, \ldots, C_n$, if X, then Y with $P < 0.05$. The $<$ sign indicates "less than." Thus this statement has a probability of being accurate all but five percent of the time. According to Reynolds, all probabilities must add up to 1.00.[14] This form not only indicates the conditions necessary for the relationship between concepts to occur, but also the degree of likelihood that the relationship will $(P = +1.00)$ or will not $(P = -1.00)$ occur. Thus the above example can be expanded: given conditions of good health (C_1), adequate diet (C_2), and reasonable amounts of rest (C_3) and exercise (C_4), if severe stress $(\uparrow X)$ occurs, then adaptation $(\uparrow Y)$ will tend to occur in proportion with a high probability $(\uparrow P)$. The abbreviated form is: C_{1-4}, if $\uparrow X$, then $\uparrow Y$ with $\uparrow P$.

Reynolds states that it is impossible to prove probabilistic statements false. Instead, to test the truthfulness of such statements, a large number of events are studied. The example Reynolds uses is to throw dice (or coins) ten thousand times to learn whether or not each side will turn up the predicted number of times.[15] For a further discussion of probability, consult other sources, such as Kerlinger.[16]

Generally, the forms of relationship statements that have just been discussed—logical, correlational or associative, deterministic, and probabilistic—tend to be used with concepts that are rather concrete and measurable. This represents an advanced state of a theory in that the relations among concepts can be readily tested through research processes—if this has not, in fact, already occurred. But there are also other forms of relationship statements that lend themselves more readily to abstract concepts. These seem characteristic of early stages of theory development.

One such is described by Hawes as the analytic form.[17] This kind of statement relates three concepts in the following manner: all of the concept X is concept Y; concept Z is X; therefore Z is Y. A more familiar presentation of this form is: "A is B; C is A; therefore C is B."[18] Or it might go like this: all men are mortal; Socrates was a man; therefore Socrates was mortal. This is called a substantive warrant in argument development of the classification type in eristic thinking (see the discussion in Chapter 4). Hawes further notes that this form is logical in nature, valid by definition, and tautological. Thus it is the basis of formal theories.[19]

As we read any theory, we believe it is wise for us to seek to identify one or more of these forms of relationships between concepts. This can readily be accomplished after identifying the major concepts of the theory and substituting X, Y, and Z for them. Mastery of this process can provide a degree of sophistication for the aspiring theoretical analyst, and it can also provide preparation for the analysis of unique and complex theories. We also need to continuously bear in mind the distinctions that are made between assumptions and relationship statements. To recap, assumptions generally provide the framework within which concepts move or change according to the pattern revealed in theoretical relationship statements.

Like statistics and numbers, which provide specific patterns of relationships between concepts within a theory, models also provide general, conceptual patterns for groups of theories. According to Fawcett, models "represent the first step in developing the theoretical formulations needed for scientific activities."[20] Models tend to develop within the creative thoughts of scholars and reflect the perspectives of the discipline. Thus Fawcett distinguishes models from theories in that models provide a "world view" of a discipline while theories focus on specific phenomena and provide detailed descriptions and explanations.[21] Models are metaphoric representations of the interaction between and among the concepts of a discipline's basic paradigm. A model's purpose is primarily heuristic in that it is a tool of communication used to develop, quide, and explain theories. Hawes states that models are relatively well-developed analogies, and that they represent theory.[22]

There are numerous examples of metaphoric and analogue models that have been and are being used today. For example, industrial leaders and scholars in some professions have used the machine as the dominant model for human beings. In more recent times, an organismic metaphoric image allows the human being to be seen as an "open, self maintaining and self regulating biological system."[23] Other symbolic models that are frequently used in many disciplines and practice professions are developmental, systemic, mathematical, and symbolic interaction models.

Another type of model is the physical model, including lifelike representations, diagrams, and pictures. One common example is the representation of carbon and oxygen molecules that is frequently seen in the chemist's laboratory. In nursing, physical models are also commonly used both for learning fundamental nursing skills and for teaching clients. Examples of these include "Mrs. Chase," the ever uncomplaining patient, and models used to demonstrate the birth process. In addition, diagrams are used to show, for example, the relationships between stressors and Man's adaptation or the concepts in

Selye's theory of stress or the relationships between and among the basic needs of Maslow's theory of motivation.[24] These models are representations of relationships between and among concepts *within* a theory and are to be distinguished from models that provide a "world view" of a discipline, described above.

In using conceptual models, there are certain assumptions that scholars and scientists make. First, it is assumed that human beings can learn about the world. Second, it is assumed that there is some order that can be imposed upon the phenomena being investigated. Third, it is assumed that all models are based on some sense of systems being in effect. And finally, it is also assumed that the model selected will be to a considerable degree bound by the scholar's culture, that the world view in vogue in the scholar's society tends to bias his or her thinking.[25]

Roy provides a conceptual model for nursing that is rather specific. She defines this model as "a set of concepts that identify the essential components of nursing practice."[26] She lists elements of this model as identified by Johnson:

1. A goal of action.
2. A descriptive term for patiency (the patient).
3. The actor's role (the nurse).
4. A source of difficulty (the patient's health).
5. An intervention focus and mode (the goal and plans).
6. Consequences, intended and unintended (desirable and undesirable outcomes).[27]

This model does not appear to be a "world view." Rather, it seems more like a shopping list identifying what is to be included in a model for nursing.

SCOPE

The heart of a theory is its statements of relationships among concepts or constructs. Because a theory *is* a system of relationship statements, any statement that describes the association and changes between concepts must be included. Research projects that add to a discipline's knowledge base are designed to test one or more relationship statements of a specific theory. Generally, statements of hypothesis are derived from the theoretical relationship statements. A hypothesis is a relationship statement that is yet to be verified through research. Then, in the research process, if data reveal sufficient support for it, the hypothesis may come to be called an empirical generalization.

When this support is "overwhelming," according to Reynolds,[28] the hypothesis or relationship statement may then be called a law. Axioms and propositions are generally so well supported by research that they are widely accepted as self-evident truth.[29] Generally, these relationship statements are used to express scientific knowledge within a discipline. Thus theoretically based research processes are instrumental in expanding the knowledge base of disciplines and practice professions such as nursing.

The process of stating relationships between concepts in a theory and the validation of these relationships has been described by Mauksch and Ketefian as existing on a continuum between theory and practice.[30] (See Figure 10.) In other words, practice-oriented disciplines exist to fulfill a social need, and ideas and questions originate at the interface of practice and social need. It is from this point of contact that ideas and questions flow backward over the continuum to stimulate the development of theories and "pure" research (research to produce new knowledge), as seen in section A of Figure 10. Some ideas and questions stimulate theory and research designed to describe, explain, predict, and control a problem of the practice context, as in section B of Figure 10. Other research studies seek to deliberately apply theories and research to specific areas of social need (section C, Figure 10). But at D in Figure 10 there is a definite break in the continuum. At this point we find the synthesis of knowledge. This represents a reorientation of the conduct of investigations, with greater emphasis on application in practice contexts in which services are delivered (sections E, F, and G in Figure 10). Thus ideas and questions arising from the interface of practice and social need "fall out" all along the continuum to serve as stimuli to scientific and scholarly activities that develop and expand a practice discipline's knowledge base.

In well-developed disciplines, the validation of relationship statements of theories through scholarly inquiry is cumulative. Here scholars and scientists develop long-term programs to investigate one theory or one problem area, and research studies are replicated to reinforce primary findings. Hans Selye's lifelong work investigating the human body's reactions to stress[31] serves as an excellent example of this sort of research, the kind of research that needs to be encouraged in nursing. Ketefian, for instance, states that new researcher roles are needed in nursing in which the nurse has "one foot in the world of research and the other in the world of practice."[32] But some barriers to the development of such a role have been inherent in the practitioners themselves as well as in the contexts of their practice. Only 15 to 20 percent of the members of the nursing profession have baccalaureate or higher de-

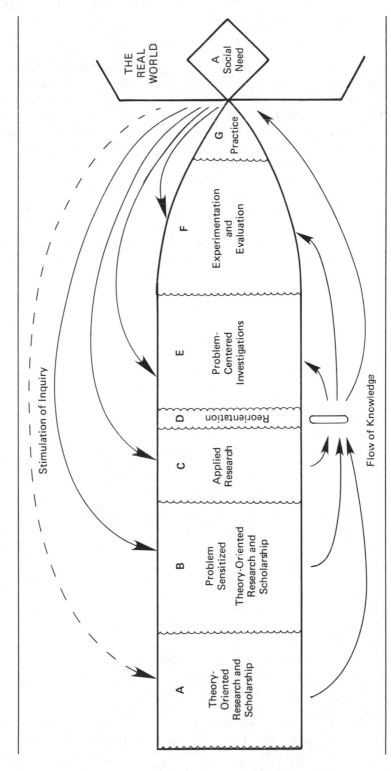

Figure 10. The theory-research-practice continuum, adapted from models by Mauksch and Ketefian.

grees, which means that a large proportion of the nurse population has not been educationally prepared even to apply new knowledge provided by research. In addition, most practice contexts are highly routinized, designed primarily to meet the needs of the organization, so that the initiative of nurses working within them is stifled. Furthermore, any initiative shown in theoretical investigations, and often even that shown in mere problem-oriented investigations, has gone unrewarded if not blatantly rejected by peers and colleagues. Thus Ketefian states that nurses in a researcher-practitioner role need the support of communication networks to maintain a climate that encourages shared theory-research values between them and other nurses in similar roles. Indeed, a number of studies have supported the positive "effects of norm setting and social controls by the scientific community on the individual scholar."[33] Apparently, the maintenance of such a value climate tends to be predictive of quality research.

Since developing relationship statements is so important in providing meaning to theory and theory testing—and thus to the development of a knowledge base for a discipline—how do we go about deliberately developing relationships between concepts? By thinking, of course. And by carefully defining concepts.

As is true of most skills, we need to practice thinking in certain ways. In Chapter 4, we discussed the six different ways of thinking that are characteristic of various disciplines, ending with a discussion of eristic thinking as a broad framework for the development of theories in nursing. In addition, skills like deductive and inductive thinking are also commonly known to most of us. However, there are even more specific patterns of thinking, which we have arbitrarily labeled "polarized," "grid," and "factoral" thinking.

After carefully defining a concept, we can think about polarized amounts of that concept on a continuum. This is called *polarized thinking*. The continuum will necessarily be concerned with amounts of the concept, since measurement is inherently important in developing relationships.

We can begin by simply identifying the low and high amounts of the concept. For example, we might use the concept, "coping."

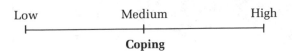

At first, we might think about how a person behaves when displaying low coping as opposed to high coping. Under low coping, a person is "laid back" and very easygoing. But that same person under high coping is quite tense, "up tight" and "spaced out." If ideas are coming easily, we might go on to identify medium amounts of this concept. For example, a person of medium coping might be described as being alert and productive.

Polarized thinking provides a description of two, and perhaps three, nominal categories that characterize the concept. In order to relate two concepts, of course, we need to go through a similar process for a second concept. For example, since we usually cope with stressful situations, "stress" would be a reasonable and logical choice for the second concept.

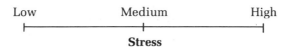

Low-stress situations can be described as quiet, calm, and peaceful, with low risk. In contrast, high-stress situations might be noisy, hectic, and turbulent, with high risk. Medium stressful situations could be described as something akin to "normal" amounts of noise and activity, with moderate amounts of risk involved.

With a second concept briefly defined, we can now move on to *grid thinking*. Here, by placing two polarized concepts at right angles to one another, we can map out a conceptual space or grid. For example, the polarized continuums of coping and stress can be arranged as in Figure 11. The space within the angle formed by the two polarized continuums can be numbered to indicate general areas of the grid. Next, we must imagine what the interactions between the two concepts would be like in each of the five areas on the grid. Thus, after noting key descriptive words in each of the areas, we can begin to develop tentative statements about each of them. And by using X to indicate coping and Y to indicate stress, we can plot the numerical or correlational patterns to develop our statements. Examples of tentative relationship statements that can be made about the relationship between stress and coping are as follows:

1. $\downarrow X$, $\downarrow Y$ = A person capable of low levels of coping tends to function well in low-stress situations.
2. $\downarrow X$, $\uparrow Y$ = A person capable of low levels of coping will tend to experience anxiety in a high-stress situation.
3. $\uparrow X$, $\downarrow Y$ = A person capable of high levels of coping will tend to be bored and lethargic or restless in low-stress situations.

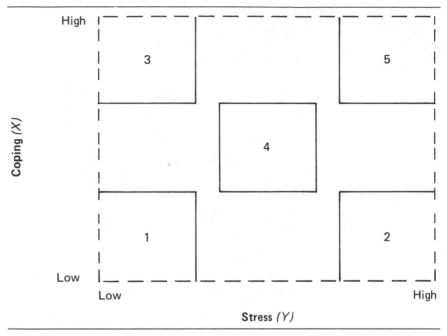

Figure 11. Grid thinking.

4. $\sim X$, $\sim Y$ = A person capable of moderate levels of coping will tend to be productive and reasonably effective in a situation of moderate amounts of stress.
5. $\uparrow X$, $\uparrow Y$ = A person capable of high levels of coping will tend to be stimulated, challenged, and productive in a high-stress situation.

Our readers may not agree with these tentative statements. In fact, some of them, and maybe even all of them, may not seem reasonable or realistic. This is expected. After all, once the statements have been derived from the correlational patterns, we still need to carefully evaluate each one of them. As potential theorists and researchers, we need to choose the statement that seems most reasonable and worthy of further consideration. It is at this point that the scholar considers whether or not he or she wishes to devote the next five years to investigating it or whether or not to seek a $50,000 research grant.

Factorial thinking merely involves adding a third (or more) concept to the pattern we've just established. Thus the correlational grid is expanded to include two or more categories of the third concept or

			Stress		
			Low	Medium	High
High	Health	Well			
		Ill			
Medium	Health	Well			
		Ill			
Low	Health	Well			
		Ill			

(Coping — vertical axis label)

Figure 12. Factorial thinking.

variable within each category of the first concepts. For example, we might add the concept of health (Z) and define it on a polarized continuum as illness versus wellness. This concept would logically characterize the person doing the coping rather than the stressful situation. Thus the factorial thinking grid would probably display the concepts as shown in Figure 12. Again, we merely speculate here about the statements that could be made concerning the interaction between the three concepts in each block on the grid. For example, one or more of the following relationship statements might be worthy of testing through research:

1. Levels of stress tend to be associated with comparable levels of coping for safe levels of health.
2. High levels of stress associated with low levels of coping tend to result in low levels of health.
3. The level of stress associated with higher levels of coping tends to occur in high levels of health.

These statements of relationship were developed by groups of nursing students and are within the nurses' statements of assumptions and specific definitions of each concept. This example represents their first effort in developing their own theory of how people, ill or well, cope in situations of varying degrees of stress.

Admittedly, these examples are somewhat general and global, but they do demonstrate the manner in which a theorist "toys" with concepts in the process of developing relationship statements within a theory. Remember that polarized thinking is just nominal counting or setting up descriptive categories within a concept. Grid thinking is looking at how two concepts vary in the presence of changing amounts of each other—hence a "variable" is another term used for a concept. An "independent variable" is the concept manipulated or changed by the experimenter, and a "dependent variable" changes depending on how it is related to (dependent on) the independent variable. Factorial thinking is derived from the statistical tools of factor analysis and the analysis of variance. These statistical tools provide methods of identifying, breaking down, and testing the statistical significance of changes or variances that come from many different sources, including those variances that are deliberately caused by the experimenter as well as those changes that arise from sources that might be uncontrollable or unknown to the experimenter.[34]

Over time, statements such as those presented above are refined, operationalized, measured, and developed. Even scholars are not all that "scholarly" at first. We need only start where we are at the moment. Just being aware of these thinking methods and considering the relationship statements of a theory is a good way to begin to understand and analyze that theory. While there may be many others, we believe that these patterns of thinking are an essential part of the scope of relationship statements.

LIMITATIONS OR EXCLUSIONS

Since we are concerned only about relationship statements associated with theories, there are a number of meanings attached to the term "relationship" that need to be set aside and separated from our present interpretation. The initial distinction to make is in differentiating relationship statements from assumptions. If these differences are not immediately clear, we suggest that you glance back to Chapter 7.

A second distinction can be made in that relating also means "to tell a story," "to recite," "to narrate," "to describe," or "to report" something we have experienced or witnessed. For example, we might tell the story of our life, or relate some amusing incident that occurred to us. These terms are not germane to our discussions about theoretical relationship statements—with two exceptions. Just as we might "describe" details of an event and "state" clearly and precisely some aspect of a story, so too do relationship statements need to describe details of an event and state clearly and precisely what happens.

Finally, a third distinction to be made is that meanings indicative of connections between people are limited in scope. While some theories do focus upon how people relate to one another, many more are concerned with relationships between objects, events, and things other than people. People are related by marriage, by blood lines, by interests, by needs, and so on. The list could be longer. Thus while theoretical relationship statements do include relationships occurring between people, theoretical statements are not limited to relationships between people, but include relationships among whatever concepts are the focus of a theory.[35]

ACCOMPLISHMENT, ROLE, AND FUNCTION

The primary function of theoretical relationship statements is to provide meaning to concepts. According to Hawes,[36] when a concept is systematically related to other concepts, meanings become more clear. In other words, the question, "So what?" is answered. For example, if an atomic reactor were to be located near a particular town, the uninformed resident might say, "So what? What's that to me?" It is only when the presence of an atomic reactor in such close proximity is considered in relation to the inherent, potential dangers of the functioning of that reactor that the future implications become evident.

Stating relationships between phenomena, events, facts, or things enables us to understand what is happening, and because of this understanding we are able to make predictions. This is the primary accomplishment of relationship statements. These statements have a major role in enabling us to be aware of potential outcomes, to plan, to implement ways and means of controlling outcomes, and, as a consequence, to be able to influence phenomena in our world.

ANALOGIES AND METAPHORS

In the discussions above, we have already used a number of analogies and metaphors. For example, we have referred to relationship statements as "maps into the abstract space" between concepts and as similar in form to statistical operations. It has also been noted that models are metaphoric representations of interactions among and between concepts. And in Chapter 7 an old-fashioned child's toy was used as an analogy to depict the relationship between assumptions, concepts, and relationship statements.

One other metaphor can be added here. A theoretical statement of relationship between two or more concepts is like the act of combining chemicals. When two or more of these chemicals interact, a new and unique substance is formed. For example, when oxygen and hydrogen, both gases, are combined in the appropriate proportions, a new substance (water), totally unlike either of the original elements, is formed. In a similar fashion, when we become aware that two or more concepts belong together in a particular relationship pattern, the novel perspective of this relationship is not easily forgotten.

AUTHORITY QUOTES

Some noteworthy comments about relationship statements have been made by scholars from numerous fields. Consider, for example, the following remarks by Hayes:

The discovery of fundamental relations that can be put into mathematical form, with formal mathematical rules like those of physics, depends upon our ability to observe the *right things* in the *right ways* under the *right circumstances.*[37]

And Cohen:

. . .science is not a knowledge of mere particulars, but rather a knowledge of the way in which classes are related.[38]

And Northrop:

The only way to get pure facts, independent of all concepts and theory, is merely to look at them and forthwith to remain perpetually dumb . . . .[39]

In comparing specific problem-oriented research and theoretically oriented research, Kerlinger states that:

Theoretical research aims are better because, among other reasons, they are more widely applicable and more general.[40]

He also defines theoretically oriented scientific research as follows:

Scientific research is systematic, controlled, empirical, and critical investigation of hypothetical propositions about the presumed relations among natural phenomena.[41]

These quotations provide some indication of how important theoretical relationship statements are to a theory and to the research designed to validate a theory.

There are also indications of change and of future directions in the comments of Kerlinger and Pedhazur. In the preface of a text devoted to multiple regression analysis, a single statistical tool, they note that research in the behavioral sciences is in the process of a

conceptual and technical revolution. It must be remembered that empirical behavioral sciences are young, not much more than fifty to seventy years old. Moreover, it is only recently that empirical aspects of inquiry have been emphasized. Even after psychology, a relatively advanced behavioral science, became strongly empirical, its research operated in the univariant tradition. Now, however, the availability of multivariate methods and the modern computer makes possible theory and empirical research that better reflect the multivariate nature of psychological reality.[42]

So this is Kerlinger and Pedhazur's view of the state of the discipline of psychology, and opinion that is now over ten years old. In comparison, students in basic nursing programs are encouraged to consider many aspects of a client's life situation. Yet upon entering graduate school, nursing students are urged to consider only two or three concepts or variables in their research projects. With the availability of multivariant analysis, perhaps future nursing students, both basic and graduate, will be able to consider multiple variables that can influence the client. Perhaps the newer statistical tools and computer software will provide fertile ground for the knowledge base of nursing to grow rapidly and develop.

SET OF ELEMENTS

As in the case of assuming and conceptualizing, we found the literature to be lacking a set of elements that describe the process of developing theoretical statements of relationship between concepts. Thus we propose the following set of five elements: identifying, combining, organizing, stating, and validating.

Identifying. Certain concepts are identified, concepts that seem naturally to go together or be regularly linked together in a phenomenon.

Combining. The identified concepts are combined with one another in order to find a pattern of change or movement.

Organizing. Eventually a pattern or form is discovered such that the concepts seem to unite into a whole.

Stating. A statement is then developed that describes the interaction among and between the concepts in such a manner that it explains, predicts, provides some potential for control, and suggests guides to action.

Testing. This total process of identifying, combining, organizing, and stating relationship statements ultimately leads to the testing experimentally of the validity of the statements. Scientific research serves as the means whereby relationship statements can be formally tested to determine the "goodness of fit" between the theoretical statements and reality.

This total process of developing and validating relationship statements within a theory emphasizes the inherent, close association between theory and research. Neither stands alone in the development of a discipline.

SUMMARY

In this chapter, we have presented an elaborate discussion of the third major element of a theory, the statement of relationship. This element has been defined according to the nine ways of defining any concept. In addition, we have discussed the development of relationship statements in many disciplines, including nursing. Considerable attention has been given to describing how we go about making relationship statements, including references to many commonly used relationship patterns from statistics and models. A set of five process elements has been proposed to sequentially describe the development of such relationship statements. In the chapter that follows, we will use the same approach to discuss the fourth element of a theory, evaluation.

NOTES

1. *Webster's New Collegiate Dictionary*, Henry Bosley Woolf, ed. (Springfield, Mass.: G. & C. Merriam, 1979), p. 968.
2. Ibid., p. 1126.
3. Ibid., p. 968.
4. Ibid.; *Webster's New Dictionary of Synonyms*, Philip B. Grove, ed. (Springfield, Mass.: G. & C. Merriam, 1968), p. 675.
5. Abraham Kaplan, *The Conduct of Inquiry* (Scranton, Pa.: Chandler, 1964), pp. 176–178.
6. Ibid., pp. 177, 172.
7. Ibid., pp. 173–174.
8. Winona B. Ackerman and Paul R. Lohnes, *Research Methods for Nurses* (New York: McGraw-Hill, 1981).

9. Donna Diers, *Research in Nursing Practice* (Philadelphia: J. B. Lippincott, 1979), p. 70.
10. Sister Callista Roy and Sharon L. Roberts, *Theory Construction in Nursing: An Adaptation Model* (Englewood Cliffs, N.J.: Prentice-Hall, 1981), pp. 2–4; Margaret Newman, *Theory Development in Nursing* (Philadelphia: F. A. Davis, 1979), pp. 9–13.
11. Leonard C. Hawes, *Pragmatics of Analoguing: Theory and Model Construction in Communication* (Reading, Mass.: Addison-Wesley, 1975), p. 30.
12. Paul Davidson Reynolds, *A Primer in Theory Construction* (Indianapolis: Bobbs-Merrill, 1971), p. 68.
13. Edward L. Wike, *Data Analysis: A Statistical Primer for Psychology Students* (Chicago: Aldine-Atherton, 1971), p. 144.
14. Reynolds, *A Primer in Theory Construction*, p. 74.
15. Ibid., p. 75.
16. Fred N. Kerlinger, *Foundations of Behavioral Research*, 2nd ed. (New York: Holt, Rinehart and Winston, 1973), pp. 94–116.
17. Hawes, *Pragmatics of Analoguing*, p. 31.
18. Ibid.
19. Ibid.
20. Jacqueline Fawcett, "A Framework for Analysis and Evaluation of Conceptual Models of Nursing," *Nurse Educator* (November-December 1980):10.
21. Ibid., pp. 10–11.
22. Hawes, *Pragmatics of Analoguing*, p. 10.
23. Rose McKay, "Theories, Models, and Systems for Nursing," *Theoretical Foundations for Nursing*, Margaret E. Hardy, ed. (New York: MSS Information, 1973), pp. 47–49.
24. Hans Selye, *The Stress of Life* (New York: McGraw-Hill, 1956); Abraham H. Maslow, *Motivation and Personality* (New York: Harper and Brothers, 1954).
25. McRay, "Theories, Models, and Systems for Nursing," p. 50.
26. Roy and Roberts, *Theory Construction in Nursing*, pp. 22–23.
27. Ibid.
28. Reynolds, *A Primer in Theory Construction*, p. 80.
29. *Webster's Dictionary*, pp. 79, 917.
30. H. Mauksch, "Summary," in *First Nursing Theory Conference*, C. Norris, ed. (Kansas City: University of Kansas Medical Center, Department of Nursing Education, 1969), pp. 97–104; Shake' Ketefian, "Problems in the Dissemination and Utilization of Scientific Knowledge: How Can the Gap be Bridged?" in *Translation of Theory into Nursing Practice and Education*, Shake' Ketefian, ed. (New York: Continuing Education in Nursing, Division of Nursing, School of Education, Health, Nursing, and Arts Professions, New York University, 1975), pp. 10–31.
31. Selye, *The Stress of Life*.
32. Ketefian, "Problems in Knowledge," p. 14.

33. Ibid., p. 21; R. Collins, "Competition and Social Control in Science: An Essay in Theory Construction," *Sociology of Education* (1968):41, 123–140; R. Corwin and M. Seider, "Patterns of Educational Research: Reflections on Some General Issues," in *The Educational Research Community: Its Communication and Social Structure*, R. A. Dershimer, ed. (Washington, D.C.: American Educational Research Association, 1970), pp. 17–67.
34. Kerlinger, *Foundations of Behavioral Research*, p. 147.
35. *Webster's New Collegiate Dictionary*, p. 968; *Webster's New Dictionary of Synonyms*, p. 675.
36. Hawes, *Pragmatics of Analoguing*, p. 30.
37. William L. Hayes, *Statistics* (New York: Holt, Rinehart and Winston, 1963), p. 46.
38. M. Cohen, *A Preface to Logic* (New York: Meridian, 1957), p. 170.
39. F. Northrop, *The Logic of the Sciences and the Humanities* (New York: Macmillan, 1947), p. 317.
40. Kerlinger, *Foundations of Behavioral Research*, p. 10.
41. Ibid., p. 11.
42. Fred N. Kerlinger and Elazar J. Pedhazur, *Multiple Regression in Behavioral Research* (New York: Holt, Rinehart and Winston, 1973), p. v.

Evaluation

10

The fourth sequential element in the process of developing a theory is evaluating the degree to which the theory is supported by research—that is, the degree to which the theory matches reality. The question of how we are to distinguish good theories from bad is a fundamental one for all disciplines, indeed for all mankind. Here we ask ourselves which theory has "scientific merit," what the goals of science are, and how we can "know" something.

Toulmin provides answers to all these questions by taking the position that the central aim of science involves any intellectual creation, and that any activities associated with explanatory ideas and ideals can appropriately be called "scientific."[1] In addition, he offers a number of arguments supporting the thesis that models of explanatory ideas and ideals change over the centuries. In Toulmin's view, "the idea of explanation is tied up with our prior patterns of expectation, which in turn reflect our ideas about the order of Nature. To sum up: any dynamical theory involves some explicit or implicit reference to a standard case of 'paradigm'."[2]

Consider, for example, Toulmin's explanation of the way our ideals of the natural order of things in relation to motion have evolved, with one ideal or perspective often providing a base for the development of the next. Thus, upon seeing the traces of a horse's harness break, Aristotle explained that the cart came to a halt because the horse stopped pulling. Galileo and Newton, having a different perspective, explained that the cart stopped because of friction, gravity, and air resistance, all of which were overcome by the horse's power in pulling. In other words, they contended that if nothing interfered, the cart would keep moving.

Other examples can also be found. For a time, people thought the world was flat and that the sun revolved around the earth. Eventually, however, the paradigm changed so that people now believe the world is round (or rather egg shaped) and that "the earth revolves around the sun along with a number of other planets. This shift demonstrates

131

Toulmin's argument that "the scientific ideas which survive are the ones which have best proved their worth, while those which have been discarded—for example, the ideas of the alchemists—can be thought of as the pterodactyls of science."[3] (Pterodactyls are an extinct order of flying reptiles; this bit of information makes the metaphor easier to understand.)

In an earlier discussion, we identified the functions of a theory as descriptive, explanatory, predictive, and prescriptive. You might, then, think that all theories could be evaluated on the basis of whether they meet all of these functions. But Toulmin states that although a theory may explain, it may not necessarily predict. For example, Darwin's theory of evolution may serve as a basis of explanation for the development of antibiotic-resistant organisms, but for a long time scientists were unable to use it to make predictions about what specific new species would appear. In contrast, Darwin's theory has been very helpful in organizing descriptions, explaining, and even guiding research in paleontological studies of the development of the horse. But it has only been with the advent of ecological studies and the development of our knowledge of genetics that some degree of predictive power has become possible using Darwin's theory of evolution—a century after that theory was first proposed. In addition, models and paradigms that seem useless in one discipline may sometimes prove to be a stimulus to significant advances in other disciplines, perhaps even during other times. As Toulmin reminds us, it is simply irrelevant to criticize earlier scientists for blindness, when the doctrines they failed to accept have no intelligible place within the theoretical framework of their time."[4]

We support this evolutionary perspective of science, agreeing with Toulmin that creative ideas, practices, and techniques are to be viewed as continually evolving and changing in accord with the social and intellectual standards and expectations of their times. With this perspective in mind, we will proceed in this chapter to define "evaluation" in the nine ways of defining any concept. We will also provide some contemporary guidelines for evaluating theories, guidelines that may be helpful in distinguishing between good and bad ones, at least for the time being.

DICTIONARY DEFINITIONS, SYNONYMS, AND DERIVATIONS

According to the dictionary, the term "evaluate" means to affix a value, significance, or worth to something by means of careful appraisal and study.[5] This is something that is not done hastily but with careful consideration. Synonyms of "evaluate" include "appraise," "rate," "assess," and "estimate."[6] These terms are probably more familiar in reference, for example, to having jewelry appraised or to having estimates made on a car for maintenance and repair services.

The word "evaluate" is derived from the French *evaluation*, meaning "back information."[7] However, current interpretations are not limited to looking backward. Rather, they often focus on the present conditions or status of the object of evaluation, and may also refer to future value or worth, as in making stock market investments.

OPERATIONAL DEFINITION

Of necessity, the process of evaluation requires a comparison of the thing being appraised with some standard or set of criteria. For example, when our car has been wrecked, we must decide the degree to which we wish (or can afford) to restore it. We may want it restored to its original state. We may, however, invest in major mechanical repairs, but decide not to repair dents or damage that does not interfere with the car's safe operation. Thus it can be seen that individuals may have differing degrees of "rigor" or strictness in applying various criteria.

In evaluating theories, a similar situation exists in that disciplines and even individual scholars may have varying degrees of rigor in applying criteria. In addition, there are many sets of criteria that can be used. Thus the evaluation of a theory involves the development of criteria that represent an ideal, a standard, a touchstone or gauge, with which any theory may be compared. Decisions are made regarding the degree to which the criteria are achieved, and these criteria are suggested by the literature of each discipline.

One example of this process is found in social psychology. Here Shaw and Costanzo[8] suggest the following criteria for theories in their discipline, criteria that may also be applicable to most theories in other disciplines. According to Shaw and Costanzo, the first necessary characteristic is logical consistency. This means that a theory needs to be internally consistent, that some of its statements do not contradict others. Second, a theory needs to agree with known data but also allow room for future observations in order to push to the farthest reaches of knowledge. Third, a theory needs to be testable. Unfortunately, the testability of theories can vary greatly. For example, Freud's psychoanalytic theory contains the concept of repression, in which something that is repressed cannot be recalled (and thus, by definition, something that is recalled cannot be repressed). There would seem, then, to be no way to refute or prove the existence of this concept. Generally, only one such incidence will refute a theory. We must remember too that a theory is never really "proved." Instead it is "accepted" on the basis of the amount of evidence that supports it.

There are other desirable characteristics of a theory, as suggested by Shaw and Costanzo.[9] First, statements of the theory need to be clear and simple. The terms used need to be readily understandable by members of the discipline, and the logic easy to follow. Second, statements of relationships need to be few in number. In other words, they need to be economical in explaining a phenomenon. Third, in order to increase the probability of its truthfulness, a theory needs to be consistent with theories that are closely related to it. Fourth, a theory needs to readily match real-world experiences. And finally, a theory needs to be useful in that it explains, predicts, and provides a basis for research, practice, or further advances in scientific knowledge.

In nursing, several scholars have identified similar criteria. For example, Newman suggests the following, which are specifically applicable to nursing.[10] First, the theory focuses on the life processes of human beings. Second, it reveals the patterns of those life processes that have relevance to health. And third, the theory concerns components that promote health.

Stevens also identifies certain "commonplaces" or factors that she uses in theory evaluation. These include "nursing acts, the patient, health, the relationship of nursing acts to the patient, the relationship of nursing acts to health, and the relationship of the patient to health."[11] Stevens also warns the reader to beware of "slogans" and to carefully differentiate "extraneous remarks" from the "essence" of theoretical nursing statements.[12]

We propose the addition of the following criteria according to the four major elements of the concept, "theory": assumptions, concepts, relationship statements, and evaluation. And in the following paragraphs, we will suggest certain questions that seem appropriate for the evaluator of nursing theory to answer.

First, the assumptions of the theory need to answer certain questions. What is a human being? And with which aspect or aspects of Man is the theory primarily concerned? Some theories focus only on physical states or on the intellectual development of one individual, while other theories may focus on both these areas for either one or several individuals.

We should also ask what degree of influence the present has in the theory in comparison to history, or past experience. If the past is assumed to have greater influence than the present, then this will influence the attention given to past rather than current data for development of a nursing care plan. Is the human being more influenced by present or by past events, traits or heredity? The answer to this question will also influence the assessment of the client and the nursing care plan.

In addition, we must consider the theoretical orientation to reality. Is it static or process? In other words, are human beings assumed to be incapable of change, or are they seen as dynamic, motivated beings capable of initiating change? This assumption indicates the degree of influence possible for nursing intervention, for if people are assumed to be unchanging, then custodial nursing care rather than supportive, educational nursing care would logically follow.

The most difficulty for evaluation arises, however, when we need to identify what asumptions have been omitted from a theory. For example, some nursing theories neglect to indicate that the environment for the theory is assumed to be limited to a hospital setting. Consequently, application of such theories would be inappropriate for a clinic or a community setting in which nurses practice.

The second criterion to be addressed in evaluating a theory concerns the matter of definition. Here we ask ourselves how many of the nine ways to define a concept has the theorist considered. How reasonable is the "leap of faith" between the concept and the operational definition? Is it clear to us what the phenomenon is that is being defined? Are the procedures for operationalizing the concept written in such a manner that the phenomenon defined can be operationalized for research purposes? To what degree is the concept measurable? Instruments and special effects required for observation of the phenomenon need to be specified. And if concepts are borrowed from other theories or are central to other well-known theories, then the theorist needs to differentiate any unique meanings of such concepts as they are used within the context of the theory that is being evaluated.

Third, there are also important aspects to be considered when evaluating the relationship statements of a theory. For example, what is the pattern used in stating the relations between concepts? To what degree does the pattern provide direction in the selection of statistical tools and thus facilitate research? To what degree do the statements explain phenomena, predict outcomes, provide meaning, and/or serve as guides to action? Relationship statements need to be converted to hypotheses for testing purposes, and the ease with which this can be accomplished tends to facilitate research. One can apply polarized and grid thinking, toying with relationships between the concepts, and, as a result of such conceptual toying, one can develop some indication of how reasonable and realistic the relationship statements intuitively seem to be.

Finally, the overall evaluation of a theory needs to include consideration of a number of factors that can be summarized by answering certain of the following key questions:

1. How parsimoniously or simply is the theory stated?
2. How wide is the theory's applicability and generalizability? How reliable and valid are the findings of research efforts to support the theory?
3. How well does the theory explain the phenomenon it purportedly is designed to cover? Are some areas left out? Are there some experiences for which the theory does not account? What are the areas of nursing in which this theory could or has been implemented?
4. Is the theory in agreement with known data?
5. Is it internally consistent or does one theoretical statement contradict another?
6. To what degree has the theory stimulated research among scholars?
7. How important is this theory to nursing and nursing practice?
8. If it is a borrowed theory, what other disciplines have used this theory and with what degree of success?
9. Who has criticized the theory and on what basis? How reasonable are the criticisms?

Thus we have presented some criteria that can be used as standards in evaluating theories from many disciplines, as well as from nursing. But we must remind you that additional criteria may become available in the future. Generally, these criteria seem most representative for theories of the social, behavioral, and biological sciences; many seem applicable to nursing, too.

SCOPE

Technically, the evaluation of a theory includes not only all theoretical statements and accompanying discussions but also all research efforts that may support or refute the theory. Our discussions about what is included in evaluation of theories will center on the parsimony or simplicity of their statement and structure, on scope, on their applicability, on their generalizability, on their agreement with known data and relevant research, and on their importance to the discipline and practice of the nursing profession.

The use of the term *parsimony* (thriftiness or simplicity) in discussing theoretical statements refers to the economical use of words in presenting a theory. Thus a parsimonious theory is simply and clearly stated so that all its meanings are explicit and the theory as a whole is easily comprehended. The structure or model of the theory may also be relatively simple, with the number of concepts involved limited only to those that are relevant and germane to the phenomena that are central to the theory. Explanations and examples are clearly identified and separated from the central theoretical statements so that we are not misled or confused by intellectual and conceptual detours or by extraneous comments about contemporary events, by stereotypes, or by personal biases. In other words, the major elements of a theory need to be explicitly and succinctly identified and stated to meet the criterion of parsimony.

The *scope* of theory evaluation also concerns the conceptual territory covered by the theory. As suggested by an earlier analogy, just as a spotlight's focus on a stage can be varied in size so that small or large areas of a scene are lighted, so a theory can focus on small or large aspects of a phenomenon. In this connection, Ellis states that "scope" refers to the number and variety of facts and concepts that are related; the more concepts, the broader the scope and hence the greater the significance of the theory.[13] She also adds that: "for nursing, the scope should be judged in terms of the generalizations and phenomena pertinent to an individual of the human species in the circumstances which cause him to be labeled by the concept *patient*."[14]

Thus Ellis seems to limit the scope of nursing theories to individuals, excluding groups. We might also, however, consider the scope of a theory to include the degree of break with current paradigms, using Kuhn's categories of paradigm uniqueness,[15] as discussed in Chapter 6. In addition, we might use the classification of theories according to levels of complexity as described by Dickoff and James,[16] also in Chapter 6.

Obviously we need to have settled on a definition of nursing (another limitation of scope) before we can evaluate nursing theories. Ellis implies this when she states that "if nursing deals with recovery of the person as well as the body, theory which directs practice must have the scope to cover both."[17] In a similar fashion, we need to have settled on a definition of the human being, particularly as the recipient of nursing care. Generally, nursing as a discipline focuses on the recipients of nursing services and on those changes occurring in the patients or clients that are known to be due to nursing interventions. Such definitions can serve as a guide to theory development as well as a means of evaluating the scope of a theory.

The *applicability* of a theory concerns its usefulness to nursing practice. Since nursing is not only a discipline but also a practice profession, it is necessary that its theories provide guidance in the decisions and actions taken by a nurse who is delivering care to a specific patient. Here we ask ourselves more questions. How easily can the clinically oriented nurse become familiar with the theory? Are clearly written summaries of the theory readily available in clinically oriented literature? Are nurses mentioning and referring to the theory when reporting or discussing aspects of nursing care plans? Affirmative answers to such questions provide some idea of how readily the theory is actually used.

The *generalizability* of a theory is closely related to its research. In other words, the theory needs to suggest populations, settings, experimental treatment variables, and methods of measuring those variables. If we are given a known subject population, setting, and so on, in research efforts to support a theory, to what degree can we transfer these research findings to the whole population? For example, psychological research using rats has historically been used to support learning and behavior theories, and the findings have been generalized to human populations. But the necessary assumption that rats and people behave in similar ways has been questioned by layman and scholar alike; for some, it simply does not seem to be a reasonable assumption. The safer way to generalize research findings is to apply these findings to people who have many characteristics in common with the research subjects. In this connection, Campbell and Stanley identify the generalizability of a theory as a question of external validity in research design, and they provide help to the theorist and researcher in eliminating or controlling such jeopardizing factors.[18] However, research involving human subjects presents unique problems in awareness, motivation, bias, and ethics. Thus Adair provides helpful discussions and guidelines in research design for psychologists who are involving human subjects in experiments.[19] In nursing, a similar reference would be helpful because it is logical that most of the research in nursing would need to involve human subjects, particularly those having health problems.

In discussing generalization, we need to realize that our focus so far has been on "actual" generalization as opposed to "potential" generalization. As Chinn and Jacobs explain it," 'Actual generality' refers to generality in theory that has empirical support, whereas 'potential generality' refers to theory that is broad in scope but untested in reality."[20] At the present time, most nursing theories seem to have only "potential generality" since there are limited numbers of research studies designed to test specified theoretical statements on one theory. However, during the next decade, long-term research programs designed to test specific theories will probably become common.

For a theory to have potential merit, its assumptions and statements of relationship also need to show *agreement with known data and contemporary knowledge, to be intuitively good.* It seems wise to develop an intuitively good theory about which nothing or very little is known and to initiate research projects to support it. However, to develop a theory that is intuitively unsupported is seen as a way of achieving professional infamy and scholarly suicide. Theories need to have "goodness of fit" with our perception of reality to be worthy of our research efforts. Indeed, some theories have a short life span, as it were, because, like being the "fastest gun in the West," a widely accepted "good" theory is continually in danger of being "shot down" by a better one.

Even long-standing theories can suddenly lose favor. For example, people long believed that it was foolish for humans even to try to fly, yet historical documents reveal repeated efforts to achieve this capability. Now flying is commonplace for many. Another example can be found in physics. In Athens, Aristotle proposed that all matter consists of earth, air, fire, and water. In the fifth century, Democritus, another Greek, proposed that all matter consists of small bodies that he called "atoms." This theory was forgotten, and Aristotle's held for over two thousand years. In 1543, Copernicus supported the atomic theory through his discoveries and through his own theory that the sun is the center of the universe. But once again, this theory was not accepted, and again it was set aside. In 1610, Galileo developed the telescope and discovered more data that was consistent with Copernicus' theory. He published his work in Italian rather than in the usual scholarly Latin, and more people learned of the theory that the sun is the center of the universe. Unfortunately, Galileo's teachings contradicted the religious beliefs of the Church at that time, and as a result he was held under house arrest by the Inquisition, an investigative arm of the Catholic Church. Eventually, of course, he and his predecessors were vindicated by scientific research, and today most people share their beliefs.[21] From this we can see that new theories and ideas are often rejected initially. Thus the theorist is sometimes reluctant to allow reports of his or her work to be published. Such works are often published posthumously. But in order to have potential merit, any theory needs to account for known data and propose a unique perspective or alternative explanation for the phenomena observed.

In most practice-oriented disciplines, there are two perspectives on the *relevancy of research*. For most disciplines, research that has the highest degree of relevance involves studies that are derived directly from theoretical statements of relationship. The operationalization of concepts, the target subject groups, and the contexts to be used in research design are all suggested by the theoretical statements. Typically, a series of projects is designed so that a long-term research program will systematically investigate specific relationships among concepts. Given adequate funding, scholarly interest, and continued validation of the theory by research findings, the program is continued until all relevant ideas are explored. This requires dedicated and committed scholars who are willing to devote a major portion of their careers to a particular research question.

From another perspective, however, research that is most relevant for disciplines that are also practice professions focuses primarily on the point where practice impacts upon a social need. Thus research about nurses, who they are, their length of practice, their ages, and other descriptive information is not relevant to the development of new knowledge for a discipline, despite the fact that it is necessary and important to have such data about any group of professionals. In other words, theoretically relevant research primarily involves investigations based on nursing theory and is focused on nursing practice.

Finally, another general criterion for evaluation is *the importance of the theory to the discipline and practice profession*. Specifically, the more significant theories are those that contribute to the goals of the discipline of nursing, and, in the case of nursing, the social need this practice profession seeks to fulfill. Ellis states it this way:

What is significant for nursing, what theory, what knowledge the professional nurse should spend time pursuing, is that which pertains to practice. Generation of knowledge for the sake of knowledge is not the raison d'etre for the profession of nursing—nursing is.[22]

Thus those theories that will be of significance and of consequence to nursing practice will be those which propose goals that are congruent with the goals of nursing. Such theories will have weight and influence in nursing practice.

Chinn and Jacobs note that many judgments in nursing practice are made without overt explanation based on theory, but rather are based on common practice and custom. In time, these practices and customs can be validated or replaced through the application of theories. However, Chinn and Jacobs caution that although the goals of a theory and nursing practice may be congruent, there still remains a need for wisdom and judgment in applying theories to specific situations.[23]

For example, nurses in an obstetrical unit recently became knowledgeable about the humanizing theory and practices concerning mother-infant bonding immediately after birth. In a short time, a "policy" was established that the nursing care of all new mothers and infants should include bonding practices and experiences. All went well until an unwed, pregnant teen-ager arrived from a local agency that provides protective care for such individuals. After extensive investigation, counseling, and planning, the social worker and others at the agency had encouraged and supported the teen-ager's decision to give up the baby for adoption, since she had no means of providing for the child and had been rejected by her family. During her pregnancy and residence at the agency, arrangements had been made for her to complete high school and learn computer-card keypunching. After delivery she was not to see the baby so it would be easier for her to give it up. Yet in spite of the social worker's request, the nurses insisted on using the bonding process because the practice had become a customary part of nursing care in the unit and thus mandatory. Unfortunately, the teen-aged mother's distress was only heightened by this practice, and her socio-emotional problems compounded. Clearly, the application of "humanizing" theory in this particular situation had a "dehumanizing" effect. So, in our rush to put theories into the practice of nursing, we need to consider carefully the appropriateness of a theory's application to specific situations.

Considerable attention is given to the evaluation of theories in contemporary nursing literature. And in it several processes or schema for theory evaluation are presented. Particularly noteworthy are those of Ellis, Hardy, Stevens, Duffey and Muhlenkamp, and Chinn and Jacobs.[24] The quality of theories is of continuous concern, and we need to have criteria, apply them, and be alert to achieving and maintaining standards of excellence.

LIMITATIONS OR EXCLUSIONS

Evaluation excludes the elements of judgment because to judge someone or something assumes a superior knowledge, more experience, or a greater degree of wisdom. It also assumes some special power or capability to decide what is Truth and what is Reality. In addition, it carries the connotation of an umpire or referee whose purpose is to pronounce some final decision.

In the evaluation of theories for a discipline and practice profession such as nursing, members of this group tend to be considered as equals, all having some reasonable quality of relevant knowledge, experience, and wisdom. Thus reasonable scholars seldom claim to have superhuman powers in discerning Truth and Reality and, rather than act as judges, members of a discipline and practice profession tend to evaluate through criticism to identify merits and faults, but not necessarily the latter. Specifically, to be able to criticize a nursing theory, we assume some expertise and knowledge sufficient for the individual nurse to come to a personal decision about the significance and value of a theory to his or her own practice of nursing.

Evaluation of nursing theories is to be determined by the collective personal decisions of all members of the discipline and profession.[25] Thus the use of differing sets of criteria in the evaluation process seems appropriate and is to be expected. After all, individuals may have unique criteria for specific practice needs.

ACCOMPLISHMENT, ROLE, AND FUNCTION

Evaluation generally provides three things: statements of criteria, an indication of the degree of significance, and an indication of direction for revisions. Although individuals may use their own criteria, many people hold certain criteria in common. Often their disciplines provide lists that tend to summarize these individuals' criteria. Sharing such lists through publication and through associations provides feedback to the theorist and to the user of theories as well. It tends to strengthen the disciplines and stimulate healthy competition among its members.

Shared evaluation of theories through publications, discussions, and practice provides individual nurses some indication of the degree of significance attached to a theory. For example, if one nurse expresses interest in a theory and discusses its application to practice, this tends to influence other nurses to give it more than usual consideration. And the more a theory is successfully used in clinical nursing practice, the more significant that theory becomes.

Evaluation of theories through research and, ultimately, through application provides feedback to the theorist, the researcher, and the practitioner. In this process, particular attention needs to be given not just to the merits of a theory but to criticism regarding its faults. For example, theoretical concepts such as self-actualization or self-image often are not measurable as initially defined in broad theories. However, through the revision or refinement of definitions, through methods of operationalization, or through relationship statements it may be possible to correct these faults. On the other hand, perhaps a new theory, a paradigm variation as described by Kuhn,[26] will be necessary to clear up such problems. Thus evaluation provides direction and guidance for revisions in theory, related research, and clinical application.

ANALOGIES AND METAPHORS

To be evaluated is like being disciplined. It is necessary and good because it promotes social adjustment, growth, and conformity to rules and standards. But it is also risky. To be evaluated can feel like punishment; it can be painful.

AUTHORITY QUOTES

Important quotations about the evaluation of theories have been included earlier in this chapter. However, some additional comments are worthy of attention. For example, in discussing the historical development of nursing diagnoses, Kritek states:

I contend that we have, in building nursing theories, skipped the first stage of specifying, defining, and classifying our concepts; and this has created problems. Prescriptive theory has been generated without care being given to the prior stages of theory construction. I suggest that returning to level-one theory building and doing first things first may be a worthwhile direction toward which we could redirect our energies.[27]

Another remark, from Diers, concerns nursing research, but it is also applicable to the evaluation of nursing theories:

The purpose of evaluating research is not so much to show off one's critical ability and prove what a dunce the investigator was as to evaluate the report for how well it fulfills its purposes in terms of its function for further nursing studies or for the profession in general.[28]

Dickoff and James take a strong position regarding the relationship between theory and research:

[R]esearch is not just seemingly purposeless but is in fact pointless busy work unless done not only in the context of theory but also with a clear realization of what it is that research has to say or contribute to that theory. Pure abstinence from theoretical involvement on the grounds of practical interest or research orientation may well be a defense to submerge the feelings of inadequacy or confusion surrounding the production and use of theory.[29]

From the tone of these quotations, we can sense the degree of heat that is generated by some discussions about nursing theory and research. However, some degree of heat is often necessary for growth.

SET OF ELEMENTS

As in the case of assuming, conceptualizing, and relating, we found the literature lacking in a set of elements that describes the process of evaluating theories. Thus, to complete the defining of the concept "evaluation" we propose the following set of process elements: standardizing, analyzing, appraising, and reporting.

Standardizing. Here the criteria that serve as the touchstone of the evaluating process are first identified and stated.

Analyzing. The theory itself is separated into categories or elements according to a systematic plan. Specific aspects—such as assumptions, concepts, relationships, and evaluation—are identified, classified, and appraised according to internal criteria.

Appraising. Finally, the theory in toto is appraised according to general external criteria to establish a summary statement of its significance and value.

Reporting. A written record of the evaluation process and the resulting appraisal is developed and presented, usually in formal, public statements for consideration by members of the discipline and practice profession.

This total, ongoing process of theory evaluation provides significant feedback to validate to varying degrees the work of the theorist.

SUMMARY

In this chapter we have presented an extensive discussion of the fourth element of a theory, the evaluation, according to the nine ways to define any concept. Adopting an evolutionary perspective, references were made to the works of authors from numerous disciplines as well as nursing. Considerable emphasis was focused on identifying criteria for evaluating theories as well as on the use of those criteria. References were made to the numerous sets of criteria available in nursing and related disciplines, and a set of four process elements was proposed to sequentially describe the evaluation process. In this chapter we have also presented directions and examples of the theory analysis framework proposed for use as the basis for analyzing any theory—assumptions, concepts, relationship statements, and evaluation. This analysis framework is explained and its applications exemplified in the chapters that follow.

NOTES

1. Stephen Toulmin, *Foresight and Understanding: An Enquiry into the Aims of Science* (New York: Harper & Row, 1961), pp. 57–58.
2. Ibid., pp. 79–80.
3. Ibid., p. 82.
4. Ibid., p. 95.

5. *Webster's New Collegiate Dictionary*, Henry Bosley Woolf, ed. (Springfield, Mass.: G. & C. Merriam, 1979), p. 392.
6. *Webster's New Dictionary of Synonyms*, Philip B. Grove, ed. (Springfield, Mass.: G. & C. Merriam, 1968), p. 301.
7. *Webster's Dictionary*, p. 392.
8. Marvin E. Shaw and Philip R. Costanzo, *Theories of Social Psychology* (New York: McGraw-Hill, 1970), pp. 12–14.
9. Ibid.
10. Margaret Newman, *Theory Development in Nursing* (Philadelphia: F. A. Davis, 1979), p. 2.
11. Barbara J. Stevens, *Nursing Theory: Analysis, Application, Evaluation* (Boston: Little, Brown, 1979), p. 11.
12. Ibid., p. 12.
13. Rosemary Ellis, "Characteristics of Significant Theories," in Margaret E. Hardy, ed., *Theoretical Foundations for Nursing* (New York: MSS Information, 1973), p. 81.
14. Ibid.
15. Thomas S. Kuhn, *The Structure of Scientific Revolution* (Chicago, University of Chicago Press, 1962).
16. James Dickoff and Patricia James, "A Theory of Theories—A Position Paper," *Nursing Research* 17 (1968):197–203; James Dickoff and Patricia James, "Researching Research's Role in Theory Development," *Nursing Research* 17 (1968):204–206. Also published in Catherine C. H. Seaman and Phyllis J. Verhonick, *Research Methods for Undergraduate Students in Nursing*, 2nd ed. (New York: Appleton-Century-Crofts, 1982), pp. 126-127.
17. Ellis, "Characteristics of Significant Theories," p. 82.
18. Donald T. Campbell and Julian C. Stanley, *Experimental and Quasi-Experimental Designs for Research* (Chicago: Rand McNally, 1966), pp. 5, 17.
19. John G. Adair, *The Human Subject* (Boston: Little, Brown, 1973).
20. Peggy L. Chinn and Maeona K. Jacobs, *Theory and Nursing: A Systematic Approach* (St. Louis: C. V. Mosby, 1983), p. 140.
21. Jay M. Pasachoff and Marc L. Kutner, *Invitation to Physics* (New York: W. W. Norton, 1981), pp. 3, 30–31.
22. Ellis, "Characteristics of Significant Theories," p. 89.
23. Chinn and Jacobs, *Theory and Nursing: A Systematic Approach*, pp. 174–176.
24. Ellis, "Characteristics of Significant Theories"; Margaret E. Hardy, *Theoretical Foundations for Nursing* (New York: MSS Information, 1973), pp. 18–21; Stevens, *Nursing Theory*, pp. 49–68; Margery Duffey and Ann F. Muhlenkamp, "A Framework for Theory Analysis," *Nursing Outlook* 2 (September 1974):571; and Chinn and Jacobs, *Theory and Nursing: A Systematic Approach*, pp. 131–145.
25. *Webster's New Dictionary of Synonyms*, pp. 200, 302, 475.
26. Kuhn, *The Structure of Scientific Revolution*. Also discussed in Paul

Davidson Reynolds, *A Primer in Theory Construction* (Indianapolis: Bobbs-Merrill, 1971), pp. 21–43.

27. Phyllis B. Kritek, "The Generation and Classification of Nursing Diagnosis: Toward a Theory of Nursing (1978)," in Mija Kim and Derry Ann Moritz, eds., *Classification of Nursing Diagnosis: Proceedings of the Third and Fourth National Conferences* (New York: McGraw-Hill, 1982), p. 27. Reprinted from *Image* 10 (June 1978):33–40.

28. Donna Diers, *Research in Nursing Practice* (Philadelphia: J. B. Lippincott, 1979), p. 272. See also Cheryl B. Stetler and Gwen Marram, "Evaluating Research Findings for Applicability in Practice," *Nursing Outlook* 24 (September 1976):559–563.

29. Dickoff and James, "Researching Research's Role in Theory Development," pp. 204–206.

THREE

Theory Analysis

In this section, the four elements that we have proposed to constitute a theory and have defined in the preceding chapters are now used as the basis for a systematic theory analysis. Students of any discipline are frequently asked to comment on the theories of that discipline. In order to make sensible, reasonable statements and establish ourselves as creditable and reliable members of our discipline, we need to be familiar with particular theories and be able to compare them with other, often conflicting theories. In this process it is very helpful to have a set of common elements for comparison.

Theorists in any discipline often write from different perspectives, so we must often search for commonalities as we read various theories. We also need to be discriminating since writers sometimes seem to pad theory papers with so many applications and supplemental commentaries that we can easily become lost. However, a set of common elements can serve as a guide both for the novice and perhaps even for the more sophisticated scholar.

In Chapter 11, we will present such a plan of analysis. In doing so, we are not proposing that it is the only method, or even the best one, but we offer it as a relatively easy introduction to theory analysis. After using it for a while, it will be easy to incorporate other methods of analysis into your *analysis format.*

Each discipline tends to have a basic paradigm. A paradigm sets up boundaries for a discipline, establishes goals and purposes, and gives general direction for looking at phenomena.[1] In nursing, the consensus of scholars seems to agree on the paradigm shown on page 148. Here the four major concepts of a nursing theory are the client or human being, his or her health, the environment in which the client exists, and the nurse. It is assumed that the client has a health prob-

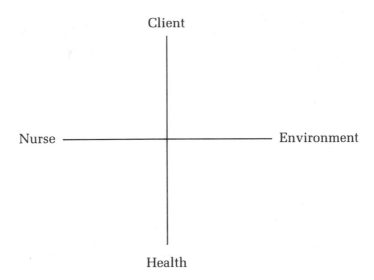

lem requiring the unique and specific knowledge and skills of the nurse. It is also assumed that the nurse intervenes to influence or change in one, two, or all three concepts in such a manner that the health of the client improves. Nursing theories are concerned with how the nurse goes about doing this influencing and changing so that we have a description of the process; can explain it; can control when, where, and how often it happens; and can predict outcomes given the specific situation to which the theory applies.

Moving from this basic paradigm, each discipline's theories tend to present unique models that incorporate all the concepts in the basic paradigm but select particular aspects to be highlighted in the theory. Each theory, then, represents an effort by one member to tell other members of the discipline how he or she thinks events happen among and between concepts in the basic paradigm.

Often theories can be grouped according to the models or "world views" used in presenting them. According to Johnson, three such models now being used in nursing are the developmental, the systems, and the interaction models.[2] Examples of the developmental model that have been borrowed from other disciplines include Erik Erikson's theory of the ages and stages of Man, Freud's psychoanalytic theory, and Maslow's theory of motivation.[3] In nursing, we have Peplau's interpersonal relationships in nursing theory.[4] Theorists from other disciplines using the general systems model include Ludwig von Bertalanffy and Anatol Rapoport.[5] In nursing, this model is used by Roy in her theory of adaptation.[6] The interaction model is derived from the communication discipline's symbolic interaction theories; examples of this include the theories of Kenneth Burke and Martin Buber.[7] In nursing, the symbolic interaction model is used in the theories of Orlando and of Wiedenbach.[8] Thibodeau identifies an eclectic model that uses two or more models. For example, Orem's theory is based on an eclectic model that includes developmental systems and symbolic interaction.[9]

A discipline's choice of models has a significant influence on the development of the knowledge base of that discipline. This is because the model that is used dictates to a great extent what questions will be asked, what kinds of events or phenomena will be observed, what research designs are to be used, what goals are to be set, and ultimately what characteristics the body of knowledge that is accumulated will have. In other words, models restrict the scholar's perspective just as our view is restricted when we pass through a tunnel. Models do give us a certain "tunnel vision."

In the chapter that follows, we will present our own plan for the analysis of theories using a number of theories as examples and for comparison. Then, in Chapter 12, Sister Callista Roy's adaptation nursing theory will be analyzed as representative of the systems model. The symbolic interaction model will be represented in Part Four by an in-depth analysis of Duldt's theory of humanistic nursing communication.

For those who wonder how a particular model or conceptual system is selected as appropriate for a discipline, Johnson suggests certain criteria.[10] One is "social congruence," which means that the expectations of society are fulfilled through the application of a theory based on a particular model. Another, "social significance," requires that the results of applying the theoretical model lead to important outcomes for the client. Finally, "social utility" requires that the theoretical model give definitive direction for practice, education, and research within the discipline. Johnson further states that "truth" is not involved in selecting models for disciplines like nursing. Rather, such a selection is a social decision, judged by society at large according to criteria beyond the model and beyond the discipline itself. Thus nursing scholars take the risk of believing that nursing as a discipline and a profession does have a unique service to offer and seek to prove this belief by meeting society's criteria through the development of models and theories. However, Johnson cautions that "none of these models can be judged at this point in time as the best model, or the right one for nursing." She adds, "The scientist in nursing also faces the exciting challenge of influencing nursing's direction and progress as a profession and a scientific discipline."[11]

We urge our readers to consider the chapters in Part Three very carefully. As a member of society, you can make your own judgments. And you can also have an impact on the fundamental tenets of your chosen discipline. While many will view this period in the development of nursing as a hopeless scramble of problems, we see it as an exciting one in which to enter the profession.

NOTES

1. Janice A. Thibodeau, *Nursing Models: Analysis and Evaluation* (Monterey, Calif.: Wadsworth Health Sciences Division, 1983), p. 2.
2. Dorothy E. Johnson, "Development of Theory: A Requisite for Nursing as a Primary Health Profession," in Norma L. Chaska, ed., *The Nursing Profession: Views Through the Mist* (New York: McGraw-Hill, 1978), p. 213.
3. Erik H. Erikson, *Childhood and Society*, 2nd ed. (New York: W. W. Norton, 1949); Sigmund Freud, *An Outline of Psychoanalysis* (New York: W. W. Norton, 1949); and Abraham H. Maslow, *Motivation and Personality* (New York: Harper and Brothers, 1954).
4. Hildegarde Peplau, *Interpersonal Relations in Nursing* (New York: G. P. Putnam's Sons, 1952).
5. Ludwig von Bertalanffy, "An Outline of General System Theory," *British Journal of Philosophical Science* 1 (1950); Anatol Rapoport, "Modern Systems Theory—An Outlook for Coping with Change," in Brent D. Ruben and John Y. Kim, eds., *General Systems Theory and Human Communication* (Rochelle Park, N. J.: Hayden, 1975).
6. Sister Callista Roy and Sharon L. Roberts, *Theory Construction in Nursing: An Adaptation Model* (Englewood Cliffs, N. J.: Prentice-Hall, 1981).
7. Kenneth Burke, *Language as Symbolic Action* (Berkeley: University of California Press, 1968); Martin Buber, *I and Thou*, trans. by Walter Kaufmann (New York: Charles Scribner's Sons, 1970).
8. I. J. Orlando, *The Dynamic Nurse-Patient Relationship* (New York: G. P. Putnam's Sons, 1961); Ernestine Wiedenbach, *Clinical Nursing: A Helping Art* (New York: Springer, 1964).
9. Thibodeau, *Nursing Models*, pp. 43–65.
10. Johnson, "Development of Theory," p. 213.
11. Ibid., pp. 213, 214.

Analyzing a Theory

11

Now that we have defined the sequential elements of a theory, we can put this information to work by using it to analyze theories. To "analyze" means to separate the whole into its component parts in order to examine them individually and in relation to one another.[1] In this chapter, we will present an overview of an analysis process, along with some rather specific directions. For examples we will refer to several theories that should be familiar to most students of nursing theories.

THE ANALYSIS PROCESS

It is often difficult for students of theoretical analysis merely to read a theory and comprehend it without taking notes. Therefore we suggest that you use an analysis format that we'll call a theory analysis sheet. For this, obtain a legal-sized note pad on which to take notes according to the form recommended in Figure 13. As you read and identify the major elements of the theory, record these assumptions, definitions, and relationship statements in the appropriate columns. Remember to cite page numbers for later reference.

After you have carefully read the theory once and recorded information in the appropriate columns, you will have condensed the structure of the theory to about two or three pages, thus providing a panoramic view of the entire theory. Then the evaluation column can be completed as you consider *selected* criteria. It is wise to save the theory analysis sheets that you use for each theory so you can add additional information or notes as research and criticisms appear in the literature. One major advantage of this process is that it makes it easier for you to compare various theories. (For examples, see Appendix B and Appendix C.)

On the theory analysis sheet, the spaces for the name of the theorist and the theory seem self-explanatory. The name of the textbook, article, or reference is necessary for identification of the source, par-

Theorist:

Theory:

Reference:

Phenomenon Observed:

Assumptions	Concepts	Relationship Statements	Evaluation (Selected criteria)
			Parsimony
			Scope
			Applicability
			Generalizability
			Agreement with known data
			Relevant research
			Importance to discipline and profession

Figure 13. Theory analysis sheet.

ticularly after you have developed a number of theory analysis sheets. However, the rest of the sections of the sheet need a bit of clarification.

The Phenomenon Observed

The *phenomenon observed* refers to what it is that the theorist is attempting to explain. "An observable fact or event of scientific interest susceptible to scientific description and explanation" is generally the dictionary definition that is given for the term "phenomenon."[2] In other words, it is a "happening" in reality that is not initially understood.

We can cite a number of examples of the sort of phenomena that are observed by well-known theorists outside the field of nursing Maslow, for instance, seeks to explain motivation, the force that moves people to act the way they do, and proposes that his theory is applicable to all human beings.[3] In contrast, Erikson looks at the phenomenon of the psychosocial development of human beings of all ages in the United States, and Piaget studies the intellectual development of children but not adults.[4] Thus each theorist identifies and specifies the phenomenon, event, or "territory" that he seeks to clarify, describe, and explain. This phenomenon is usually identified early in the theoretical discussion and needs to be kept clearly in mind as the reader proceeds through the theory.

Turning to nursing theories, similar unique ways of viewing phenomena can be identified. For example, Travelbee, in her theory of the interpersonal aspects of nursing, looks at the nurse-patient relationship. In other words, she does not consider physical care or treatment, but only the way in which nurses and patients interact interpersonally.[5] In contrast, Yura and Walsh study the total nursing process.[6] Thus, the "territory" Travelbee includes in her theory is encompassed by that of Yura and Walsh.

Assumptions

We have defined an assumption, briefly, as a statement that is arbitrarily or tentatively accepted as being true without proof. These may be recognized as descriptive statements of the way things do not "move" or change, but at the same time they have implications for relationships among the concepts. For example, we might assume that the floor is made of Swiss cheese. Having made that assumption, we might think of its implications—about how it would change our habits of walking. Thus the assumptions we make have implications for the content of the theory.

The differences in the assumptions of nursing theories can also be identified. For example, Travelbee assumes that what a nurse believes about the nature of human beings profoundly influences her ability to relate to clients.[7] She also assumes that although human beings are more different than alike, they are alike in that all have basic needs. In contrast, Yura and Walsh provide a specific way of perceiving human beings—that they have worth and dignity, and that they have needs that must be met.[8]

Nursing theorists tend to state some premise about human beings, nurses, patients, and the environment. These assumptions may be general in nature or they may set up specific boundaries. However, we must be alert to other topics about which theorists may make assumptions. Typically, these assumptions, whatever the topic, are analogous to the "stage" upon which the concepts or "actors" and the "lines" they speak or the relationship statements seem to come alive.

Concepts

A concept is a thought or notion that is related to a symbol, term, or word. A concept labels the total phenomenon, as in Maslow's "motivation," Travelbee's "interpersonal aspects," or Yura and Walsh's "nursing process."[9] Usually there are at least two concepts in a theory, and often there are many more.

It is also helpful to look for sets of elements for the theorist's concepts—in other words, to categorize or classify the parts of a concept. Not all theorists use sets, so don't be distressed if you can't find any. However, it seems to us that most theorists who use eristic thinking do develop sets for concepts. For example, Maslow's major concept, motivation, has a set of elements that are developed according to the theme of human needs—physiological needs, safety, love, recognition, and self-fulfillment.[10] In Erikson's theory of the psychosocial development of human beings, the major concept, socialization, has a polarized set of elements that are developed according to the increasing levels of complexity of social interactions achieved at increasing stages or sets of ages—trust versus mistrust, autonomy versus shame, initiative versus guilt, industry versus inferiority, identity versus role confusion, intimacy versus isolation, generativity versus stagnation, and integrity versus despair.[11] The polarization of this set—or sets, if you prefer—contributes to Erikson's special way of relating these elements or subconcepts. This successful achievement tends to result in the positive element (trust, autonomy, and so on) and failure to develop tends to result in the negative (mistrust, shame, and the like). We need not, then, expect a single, neat set of elements, but may discover other unique, meaningful arrangements.

The concepts of "nurse," "health," and "illness" are used by Travelbee as well as by Yura and Walsh.[12] However, Travelbee also uses the concepts "human being," "patient," "communication," "suffering," and "relationship." Furthermore, Travelbee views the human being as having two major elements or subconcepts: nurse and patient. In contrast, Yura and Walsh do not use "human being," but use "nurse" and "client." The difference is subtle but important. Travelbee sees a human being as having special characteristics of "humanness" that she applies to the nurse and the patient alike. Thus there is a certain equality in sharing these characteristics in common. In contrast, Yura and Walsh seem to set the nurse apart from the client, seeing the nurse relating to the client in a programmed manner, applying client-centered care. In their theory, the nurse is the helper and the client the recipient. Thus the relationship described does not stress equality.

Other differences can be identified in the theorists' definitions of other concepts. For example, Travelbee's concept for contact between the nurse and patient is "relationship," meaning feeling, thinking, acting, and perceiving together (another set). Yura and Walsh use "nursing process," which means assessing, planning, implementing, and evaluating (still another set); it is through this process that, for Yura and Walsh, a nurse-client relationship is possible.

Generally, in assessing a theory it is important to identify the concepts and note not only how each is defined but also the manner in which the concept's elements are organized into sets. It is necessary to know these things in order to understand the next part of a theory, the manner in which each concept relates to the others.

Relationship Statements

Relationship statements show how two or more concepts (and perhaps subsets of concepts) are systematically associated or connected. Such statements provide meaning to a theory. Typical patterns of relationships between concepts can be easily identified if we write the letters X, Y, Z, and so on, over words that are identified as concepts. For example, correlational patterns are direct (increase X and Y increases, or vice versa) and indirect (decrease X and Y increases, or vice versa).

As we read a theory, these patterns can be noted. For example, Travelbee states that in order to establish a relationship (Y) it is necessary for us to perceive humanness (X) in others; in other words, if X, then Y.[13] Yura and Walsh state that if the nursing process (X) does not proceed sequentially (assessment, planning, implementation, and evaluation) then there tends to be limited progress toward health (Y); in other words, if no X, then no Y.[14] These are some of the patterns of relationship that can exist between concepts. Additional ones may be found in other references, such as Reynolds and Hawes.[15] A theory *is* a set of relationship statements. And such statements become hypotheses to be tested in research.

Evaluation

The evaluation of a theory is the process of trying to determine its degree of truth, or the match between relationships (hypotheses) and reality. This is also known as research. We recommend that you set up your own criteria to evaluate consistently all the theories that you study. This will tend to facilitate comparisons between theories later on.

For example, as you read a theory, note the number and quality of research studies that have been reported concerning that theory. Ask yourself to what degree the research findings support the theoretical statements. This is difficult to do because it requires a strong educational background in research, which few people have. However, for some time introductory research and statistics courses have been required for baccalaureate degrees, including nursing. Taking such courses, or reviewing notes from them, would obviously be helpful.

Unfortunately, it is difficult to evaluate nursing theories on the basis of research because very little has been done to systematically conduct such a program. This reflects the uncertain state of the discipline, but fortunately things seem to be changing.

When study results *are* available, then most research texts in the field can be consulted for detailed information about how to critique them. In this process we generally look at the manner in which the concepts are operationalized, or made to happen. For example, one researcher operationalized the concept "hunger" by noting how many crackers and how much milk college men consumed after a period of starvation. But it would seem more appropriate to nurses to take blood sugar tests several times over the period of starvation and relate these to the subjects' reports of experiencing hunger. In evaluating research, ask yourself whether or not the manner in which the concept is made to happen makes intuitive sense to you.

Also look at the subject group that has been chosen to be included in the research. Is this group representative of the group of people with whom the theory is concerned? How appropriate are the statistics that have been used? Could the researcher have influenced the results in some manner through inappropriate data collection procedures? These and other similar questions provide valuable feedback to the theorist.

Nurses are particularly fortunate in that providing feedback to theorists in their field is both realistic and possible. Many nursing theorists speak at major regional or national nursing conventions and meetings; their addresses and phone numbers are readily available. This makes direct, personal contact with nursing theorists possible for all, thus providing a vital part of the growth and acceptance of theory development about nursing.

As a practical matter, it is sometimes difficult to decide which of the theorist's publications is most appropriate to use as the basis of theory evaluation. Often we must simply exercise our own judgment. For example, if the theorist has written one rather complete, formal statement of the theory, either in an early or recent publication, then it would seem most appropriate to use only the one reference as the primary source for analysis. In nursing, however, some theorists have published a number of articles and books that reveal the development of a theoretical perspective, without the publishing of a formal statement. In this event, we would probably consider the most recent publications as primary sources, assuming them to be the most complete and ultimate statements of the theorist.

SUMMARY

In this chapter we have described a way of analyzing theories, particularly theories that arise from disciplines that use the eristic mode of thinking. Examples of theories relevant to nursing have been used, as well as two nursing theories, to demonstrate each of the four aspects of this analysis: making assumptions, identifying concepts, forming relationship statements, and evaluating through research. We have suggested that as you read a theory, you take notes on these aspects on a theory analysis sheet. Thus upon completion of your reading of the theory, the basic information about it will be summarized in a reasonably succinct, organized manner. A second and third reading will then reveal further details that can be added to your initial notes.

Information for the evaluation of the theory can be entered according to whatever criteria you choose to use. After analyzing several theories in this manner, you will find similarities and differences between them that can be readily identified. In the next chapter, this process will be used to analyze one theory.

NOTES

1. *Webster's New Collegiate Dictionary*, Henry Bosley Woolf, ed. (Springfield, Mass.: G. & C. Merriam, 1979), p. 41.
2. Ibid.
3. Abraham H. Maslow, *Motivation and Personality* (New York: Harper and Brothers, 1954).
4. Erik H. Erikson, *Childhood and Society* (New York: W. W. Norton, 1950); Jean Piaget, *Six Psychological Stages* (New York: Random House, 1976).
5. Joyce Travelbee, *Interpersonal Aspects of Nursing* (Philadelphia: F. A. Davis, 1966).
6. Helen Yura and Mary B. Walsh, *The Nursing Process: Assessing, Planning, Implementing, Evaluating*, 2nd ed. (New York: Appleton-Century-Crofts, 1973).
7. Travelbee, *Interpersonal Aspects of Nursing*.
8. Yura and Walsh, *The Nursing Process*.

9. Maslow, *Motivation and Personality;* Travelbee, *Interpersonal Aspects of Nursing;* Yura and Walsh, *The Nursing Process.*

10. Maslow, *Motivation and Personality.*

11. Erikson, *Childhood and Society.*

12. Travelbee, *Interpersonal Aspects of Nursing;* Yura and Walsh, *The Nursing Process.*

13. Travelbee, *Interpersonal Aspects of Nursing.*

14. Yura and Walsh, *The Nursing Process.*

15. Paul Davidson Reynolds, *A Primer in Theory Construction* (Indianapolis: Bobbs-Merrill, 1971); Leonard C. Hawes, *Pragmatics of Analoguing: Theory and Model Construction in Communication* (Reading, Mass.: Addison-Wesley, 1975).

A Theory of Nursing: A Systems Model **12**

In this chapter we shall present a discussion of the systems model and an analysis of a theory that is based on it. The theory in question is Roy's theory of adaptation, which Johnson has identified as an example of the systems model applied to a nursing theory.[1] In our discussion we will first present a brief description of the systems model and a few comments to introduce the theorist, Sister Callista Roy. Next her adaptation theory will be analyzed according to the four major elements of a theory: assumptions, concepts, relationships, and evaluation. The theory analysis sheet in Appendix B summarizes the published information about Roy's theory, using her latest book as the primary source.[2] This analysis provides one example of the process that was proposed in the preceding chapter.

THE SYSTEMS MODEL

Historically, the general systems model arose out of an increasing concern about the overspecialization of most disciplines. In the 1950s, the scientific world seemed very segmented, and specialists appeared to be increasingly unable to communicate across the disciplines. Thus a way was needed of looking at general phenomena in many disciplines—a world view. In other words, a deductive, predictive, and heuristic model was needed to offer a new view of phenomena in order to gain a greater understanding of the whole.·

The general systems way of thinking grew out of these concerns and needs. However, some have yet to decide if it is a theory, a philosophy, a world view, or some combination of the three.[3] Nevertheless, Laszlo states that it is a philosophy based on the assumption that "thinking about man and the world in terms of systems is not to force the facts of experience into the Procrustean bed of a preconceived abstract scheme, but rather is warranted by the applicability of systems concepts to many spheres of inquiry."[4] Thus individual theories can be used as points of reference within the broad, general scope of the systems model.

A group of assumptions are generally made by scholars when using the systems model. First is the notion of the wholeness of organisms, organizations, and organized complexities.[5] Second is the agreement that a multi-individual unit is more than the sum of its parts. Third is the assumption that causation arises from many levels within a system, between systems, and between systems and the environment. Fourth, it is assumed that one set of circumstances or conditions can lead to different outcomes; in addition, differing initial circumstances or conditions can result in a single outcome. Fifth, it is assumed that information-processing systems move data through networks from one place to another, and that communication processes involve the functional use of data.[6]

The systems model recognizes that there are apparent similarities of structure in the phenomena of different fields, and that reality is probably highly organized and complex. Therefore it is proposed that some degree of integration of the natural and social sciences is possible, particularly in the nonphysical sciences, by identifying common principles and patterns of systems that commonly appear in theoretical statements across various disciplines.[7] An important and relevant focus of the general systems model is upon living organisms, which are viewed as "open" systems, maintaining life at a "steady state" through continuous inflow-outflow processes, through organization, hierarchy, and an ordered wholeness.[8] Since nursing is concerned with the human being as a living organism and with the maintenance of health (a "steady state"), this model can readily be applied to the development of nursing theory.

It has been noted earlier that the "world view" models used in a discipline dictate the questions that are asked. Thus the systems model leads the theorist to ask about the processes in input and output of individual systems. In using it, we seek to determine how parts function interdependently to maintain a whole. We become concerned about the nature of the information-processing and of the communication systems within the individual unit as well as with other systems and the environment. We also focus on how and why change occurs, and what processes are involved in maintaining a "steady state." Since the survival and maintenance of the system is central to the systems model, such a model is readily applicable to nursing. After all, if we view the patient or client as a system, then the generally accepted goal of nursing—to assist in maintaining health and to help cope with changes due to illness—can be restated. Our goal now is to assist the human system in maintaining a steady state.

The scope of the systems model is very broad. Generally, a system consists of a whole with interdependent parts: input of information, internal control or processing mechanisms, output, and a feedback process that maintains a steady state. The feedback and control processes function like the thermostat of a furnace, except that the control process for living systems has variable settings. As a consequence it is adaptable rather than fixed, like the furnace settings.

Systems can also be open or closed. Open systems involve matter and energy that is organized by information processing or by communication. There is an exchange with the environment of open systems, and there are input and output metabolic processes that maintain life through continually building up and breaking down components to maintain the system in equilibrium, or a steady state. There also is a corresponding increase in organization or patterning. Negentropy is the term for the increasing complexity with which open systems are capable of interchanging with the environment. Closed systems are mechanistic in nature; thus the energy within the system tends to run down like a car battery. This running-down process is called entropy, and it ultimately results in disorder, disorganization, randomness, and lack of patterning in the organization of the system. Subsystems are sets of parts or elements that constitute the whole system and work interrelatedly to achieve the goal of that system. A suprasystem is the next higher level in which a system exists, as Man exists in the environment. Each system has boundaries or outer edges that hold the elements of the system together and through which matter, energy, or information is excluded or admitted.[9]

The phenomena to be observed in the systems model include individual units in both living and non-living systems. Analogies can readily be made to the human being as a system consisting of numerous subsystems. Thus the model easily includes nursing phenomena, as well as those of most of the behavioral and social sciences.

Because of the recognition of complexity in systems, the research designs used involve numerous concepts and thus are also complex. The statistical tools analysis of variance and multivariant analysis are most appropriate. These research methods are highly advanced and probably not available to most nurses; thus significant strides in research using the systems model may be a long time coming in this field. However, the systems model is a process one rather than a linear one. And Smith proposes that process-oriented models allow for more options.[10] First, quality of the data is determined more by its "richness in explanation" than by its "objectivity." Second, Smith notes that in process-oriented models the observers' perspective or biases need to be described along with the findings. Third, explanations can be expected to differ from varying views. Fourth, because of the element of change, differing explanations from one viewpoint to another may be acceptable in differing contexts. Fifth, Smith states that the use of more holistic views will tend to develop more complete explanations. And finally, Smith notes that currently suspect research designs and methods may be accepted with this model.[11]

Models used in a discipline also influence the characteristics of the knowledge base that is developed. Thus since hierarchy and complexity are assumed, the theories and knowledge generated within the systems model will probably tend to be hierarchical and complex. Its elaborate conceptual schemes often involve concepts, sets of elements, subsets, sub-subsets, and so on. And the knowledge gained through it can be characterized by taxonomies or classifications not unlike the elaborate classification system of the biological sciences. A basic set of relationship statements can be applied to groups of major concepts of a theory as well as to the respective sets and subsets of conceptual elements. The systems model functions as an analogy in many contexts and situations. Hawes states that it is the patterning that gives meaning, and the systems model is a form of patterning.[12]

The systems model is often displayed as a group of circles to denote continual process and change, as in Figure 14. It is characterized by ordered wholeness, self-stabilization, self-organization, and hierarchism. These characteristics, according to Laszlo, promote "systemic endurance in a dynamic universe."[13]

Overall, then, it would seem that the systems model might have a releasing effect on nursing scholars in that it allows more research design options. One of its particular attractions to nursing is its facilitation of holistic views, which are currently very desirable in nursing and health care generally.

THE THEORIST

The originator of the adaptation nursing theory is Sister Callista Roy, a Catholic nun who has concentrated her efforts in nursing education since completing her doctoral work at the University of California, Los Angeles, in 1971.[14] The adaptation theory was apparently formulated during the time of her doctoral studies. While a complete statement of the theory has not been published, most of it is contained in a number of Roy's articles and books.[15] These documents indicate some shifts of perspective, but the basic concepts of the theory seem relatively unchanged. Although it is still without significant research support, the adaptation nursing theory has been used as a philosophical basis for the nursing curriculum at Mount Saint Mary's College, where Roy serves as chairman of the Department of Nursing. Roy supports the development of nursing knowledge and theories, and sees the use of

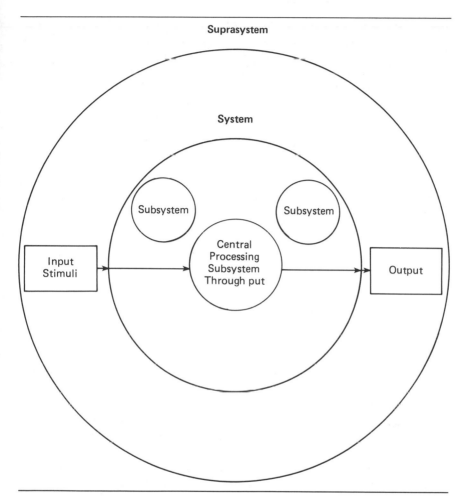

Figure 14. *The classic systems model.*

a clearly stated nursing model as essential in distinguishing nursing territory from that of other disciplines and practice professions. Because she is still relatively young, Roy will probably participate in the further development and research of the adaptation theory. She has recently served in national conference groups to study and develop nursing theories, a nursing taxonomy, and a classification system for nursing diagnosis.[16] Clearly, her work has only begun.

While Roy refers to herself as a theorist, she claims that her work on adaptation is a model, not a theory, and should not be subjected to evaluation as such.[17] However, according to our own definition of a theory and our own interpretation of the meaning of the definitions of theories commonly used in nursing, and due to the presence in Roy's work of the four major concepts of the nursing paradigm, we perceive her adaptation model to be in fact a theory of nursing. Indeed, we believe that it represents a significant contribution to nursing as a discipline and as a practice profession.

THE ROY ADAPTATION THEORY

The Phenomenon Observed

The phenomenon that Roy seeks to explain seems to be nursing practice—that is, the major elements involved in making nursing "happen." Thus her theory of adaptation seems to focus on natural ways in which human beings adapt, and mal-adapt, to a changing environment. According to this theory, nursing "happens" when a nurse does something that promotes adaptive responses for clients who have been experiencing maladaptive responses in coping with health-related concerns or problems, potential or actual.

Assumptions

While some of Roy's assumptions are stated explicitly, we have noted a few implicit ones that are important enough to be emphasized here. First, though, we must point out that Roy's theory seems to have been influenced not only by the systems model but also by physiologically based theories of adaptation such as that of Helson.[18] In fact, Roy cites numerous references to Helson's theory, as well as to other stress theories. Thus the Roy adaptation theory should be viewed as a paradigm variation of Helson's theory of stress and of the group of general systems theories.

Since it is often helpful to list assumptions according to the source of influence, we shall present Roy's assumptions according to the three major influences that we can identify: the systems model and its theories, stress-adaptation theories, and nursing.

The following assumptions seem to be derived from the systems model:

1. A system is a whole which functions as a totality due to interdependence of its parts (subsystems) for some purpose.[19]
2. Living systems are comprised of matter and energy organized by information[20] into subsystems arranged in a hierarchy.[21]

3. Information is the content (matter and energy) exchanged with the environment of a living system.[22]
4. Processing of information is communication, a necessary factor in adaptation.[23]
5. Living systems are composed of subsystems arranged in a hierarchy.[24]
6. Living systems seek to maintain balance[25] or equilibrium through an adaptive (or feedback) system of variable standards and negative feedback.[26]
7. Adaptive, living systems maintain equilibrium to ever higher levels of organization.[27]
8. A system is a process, having no beginning or ending. (Implicit)
9. Creativity is possible when the system fails and adjustments become necessary for survival of the system. (Implicit)

Those assumptions which seem to reflect the influence of stress-adaptation theories are:

10. The goals of adaptation of the total system are survival, growth, reproduction, and mastery[28] as well as high-level wellness.[29]
11. A human being is an adaptive being[30] who, rather than being a victim of the environment, has control over resources and is capable of making choices.[31]
12. In changing environments, human beings encounter adaptation problems, especially in situations of health and illness.[32]
13. Living systems are subject to stress due to internal or external stimuli or stressors.[33]
14. Living systems have an adaptation level which is the sum of three classes of stimuli: focal, contextual, and residual.[34]
15. The adaptation level of a living system establishes the parameters for positive responses to stimuli.[35]
16. Each living system must balance its use of adaptive energy. (Implicit)
17. Some stress is necessary for a living system's optimal adaptation. (Implicit)
18. Nurses can identify a client's degree of optimal adaptation and maladaptation due to excessive or prolonged stress. (Implicit)
19. Nurses can classify on a continuum of health (wellness to illness) the client's level of adaptation and maladaptation. (Implicit)
20. A living system's reaction to stress is limited to the smallest amount of adaptation necessary to maintain a steady state, and thus conserving adaptive resources or energy. (Implicit)

Assumptions that seem to reflect influences from nursing are:

21. Human beings are holistic,[36] adaptive, living systems,[37] capable of making choices and being responsible for their own bodies. (Implicit)
22. Human beings have the ability to represent reality and manipulate it for themselves and for others by spoken or unspoken words.[38]
23. The goal of nursing is to promote adaptation of human beings.[39]
24. The intended outcome of nurses' promoting clients' adaptation is high-level wellness.[40]
25. The client is an active participant in nursing care.[41]
26. Nursing interventions are directed toward manipulation of the environment.[42]

These statements seem to be the assumptions upon which Roy's nursing theory of adaptation is based. In other words, they are assumed to be true without questioning or testing.

Concepts

A theorist seldom concisely defines the concepts of a theory. Instead he or she tends to weave ideas about a concept throughout discussions and examples. This seems to be true of Roy as well. The major concepts of Roy's theory appear to include the following: "nursing," "health," "human being," "environment," and "nursing process." Several of these concepts have important subsets, which will also be defined. However, none of the definitions fulfill the requirements of the nine ways to define a term that we described in Chapter 3. Consequently, the concepts are defined here only to the extent that the theorist has developed them.

Nursing. Nursing is defined as a science, a discipline, and a health care practice. As a science, nursing is beginning to build a body of knowledge as a basis for practice. As a discipline, nursing is at the "pre-paradigm" stage, but moving toward a "common definition" of its territory. As a health care practice, nursing focuses on the assessment, diagnosis, and treatment (interventions) of clients having health problems within the domain of nursing.[43]

Health. Health is defined as a continuum[44] from illness to wellness.[45] It is determined by the client's adaptive level. "Wellness" seems to refer to stimuli or stressors falling within the zone of the client's adaptive level and thus evoking adaptive responses. "Illness" seems to refer to stimuli or stressors falling outside the client's adaptive level and thus evoking maladaptive responses.

Environment. The environment is defined as the source of external and internal stimuli. In accord with the systems model, the environment would logically consist of a suprasystem having numerous open and closed systems in its boundaries, including the open human living system,[46] as seen in Figure 15. Here we note that the human system exists within the environmental suprasystem, with subsystems$_{1,\ldots,n}$. Stimuli arise as stressors from both the external environmental supra-

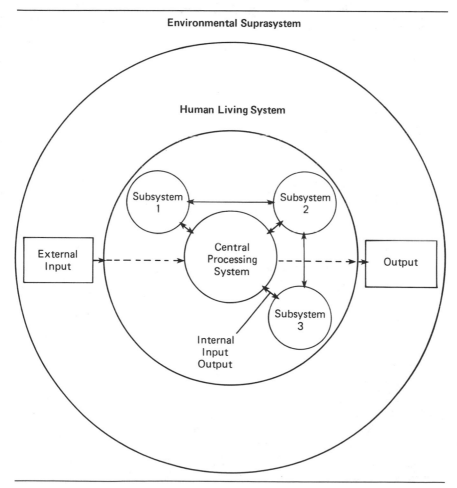

Figure 15. *An example of the systems model applied to a human being.*

system and the internal environmental subsystems$_{1,\ldots,n}$. All the systems are continually in the process of change, and each change within one system requires a corresponding adjustment on the part of adjoining supra- and subsystems.

Human being. A human being, particularly when viewed as a client or patient, is seen as an individual, family, community, or society. The principal focus, however, is upon the individual.[47] The client is viewed as an open, adaptive system receiving input from the environment, both internal and external. The totality of input is labeled stimuli. Each human being has an adaptation or tolerance level for coping with stimuli.[48]

While both nurse and client must be considered human beings, the main perspective of this theory is that of the nurse perceiving the client, who is the recipient of nursing care. Thus the nurse views the client as an open, adaptive human system continually receiving stimuli from the ever-changing external and internal environments. To maintain a balanced or "steady" state, the human system adjusts or adapts, keeping a variable adaptive level similar to that of a furnace thermostat. The human system is unique, however, in that its thermostat-like adaptive "setting" varies.

Adaptive response. The role or function of the adaptive responses is to achieve the human living system's goals of survival, growth, reproduction, and self-mastery. Effective responses achieve these goals and ineffective responses do not.[49] The adaptive responses are the human system's output.

Central processing subsystem. The human system processes all stimuli, stressors, or input through a central, or internal, processing subsystem. This system consists of two sub-subsystems, the regulator and the cognator. The regulator system consists of physiological functions of the body, and it has four sub-sub-subsystems—neural, endocrine, chemical, and "target tissue." The neural system receives stimuli, stressors, or input and stimulates the endocrine system to produce hormones or chemicals which circulate through the body to "target tissue" that responds to the chemicals.[50]

The cognator system has four sub-sub-subsystems—information processing, learning, judgment, and emotion. It generally also includes the musculoskeletal system and the psychomotor systems that produce internal and external verbalization.[51] The information system processes attention, perception, coding, and memory. The learning system processes imitation, reinforcement, and insight. The judgment system processes problem-solving and decision-making. And the emotion system processes defenses, affective appraisals, and attachments.[52] The cognator system as a whole enables the human being to grasp reality and to manipulate (change or control) it through the use of symbol systems. It is the joint effect of the interdependent functions of these sub-sub-subsystems that produces the cognator adaptive responses, both effective and ineffective. The regulator inputs into the cognator perception processes, which provide feedback to both the regulator and the cognator systems according to a systems hierarchy,[53] as seen in Figure 16.

Adaptive modes.   The human system is able to select responses from a subset of adaptive modes, or ways of adjusting to changes. These modes are labeled physiological, self-concept, role function, and interdependence. The physiological mode includes changes in fluids and

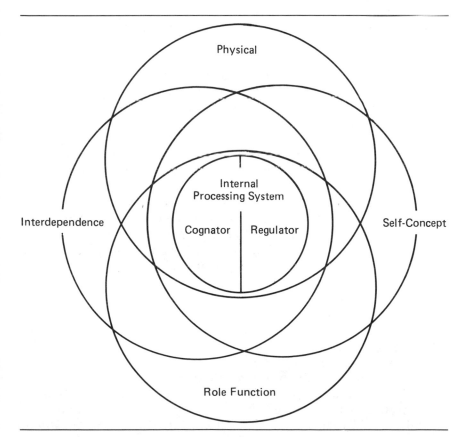

Figure 16. *Interdependent functions of the internal processing system and the adaptive modes in Roy's theory.*

electrolytes, exercise, rest, elimination, nutrition, circulation, oxygenation, and regulation of the senses, body temperature, and endocrine
states. Self-concept arises from perceptions and is one's beliefs and
feelings about himself or herself. A subset of self-concept elements
includes the physical self (sensation and body image), the personal
self (consistency, ideals, and expectations), and the moral self (ethical
beliefs). Role function refers to the part a person plays in society,
especially in dyadic, reciprocal interactions. And finally, interdependence is the relationship system a person establishes with others to
meet his or her needs of nurturance and affection, to maintain psychic
integrity, and to create interpersonal support systems.[54] These four
modes of adaptation are the effectors or activators of adaptive responses, and each is linked to the other by cognator or regulator "connectives" of the internal processing system.[55]

The adaptive modes are the total effect of three types of internal and
external input or stimuli: focal, contextual, and residual. Focal stimuli
consist of those that are of immediate concern, such as pain. Contextual stimuli consist of all other internal or external stimuli that provide a background for the experience. Residual stimuli consist of past
experiences of the regulator and cognator systems that may have an
undetermined influence on the adaptive mode.[56] The adaptive modes
are related to or communicate with the internal processor system in a
particular way. The regulator subsystem is closely associated with the
physiological mode. The cognator subsystem is associated with all of
the adaptive modes by specific inputs, pathways, and processes.[57]

The nursing process. The nurse employs a systematic method of
practice, the nursing process, to promote the client's adaptive modes
and the effective adaptation of the human system and/or to manipulate stimuli so they fall within the client's zone of adaptation.[58] The
nursing process consists of two sequential elements, assessment and
intervention.

Assessment includes data collection according to each of the four
adaptive modes and to the three levels of stimuli. Analysis of the data
leads to a nursing diagnosis, that is, an identification of (a) ineffective
adaptive modes and/or (b) stimuli that fall beyond the client's level of
adaptation. It also includes, by implication, the placement of the client's health status on the health continuum.

Drawing from the above data base, the nurse's intervention is (a) the
identification with the client of a mutually agreed upon set of goals
according to desired adjustments in the adaptive modes and/or stimuli
and (b) action taken by the nurse, that is, teaching, personal care, and
so on, to achieve the goal. Interventions, both goals and actions, are

choices or options the nurse offers the client to change the client's response potential and to bring the stimuli within the client's adaptive level.[59]

An overview of Roy's concepts. The concepts perceived to be of major importance in Roy's nursing theory of adaptation have been defined in the preceding pages. They can also be arranged in a hierarchy of sets that is consistent with eristic thinking. The following outline illustrates one method of doing so:

Nursing
Health
Human Being
    Nurse
    Client
        Adaptive Mode
            Physical
            Self-Concept
                Physical
                Personal
                Moral
            Role Function
            Interdependence
        Internal Processor System
            Regulator
                Neural
                Chemical
                Endocrine
                Target Tissue
            Cognator
                Perceptual
                Emotional
                Learning
                Judgment
Environment
    Internal Stimuli (stressors)
        Focal
        Contextual
        Residual
    External Stimuli (stressors)
        Focal
        Contextual
        Residual

Nursing Process
    Assessment
        Data Collection
        Nursing Diagnosis
    Intervention
        Goals
        Actions

The above concepts are believed to be arranged in order of importance according to Roy's theory of adaptation. Next we shall identify the ways in which Roy relates these concepts.

Relationship Statements

Relationship statements provide meaning to a theory by describing how its concepts interact. In the list that follows, the relationship statements explicitly presented in Roy's theory of adaptation are identified, along with some implicit statements we can identify.

1. If the client is an adaptive system, and if the goal of adaptation is reached when the focal stimuli are within the client's adaptation level, then nursing intervention involves manipulating focal, contextual, and residual stimuli so the person can cope with the stimuli.[60]
2. If unusual stress or weakened coping mechanisms make a client's usual attempts to cope ineffective, then the person needs a nurse.[61]
3. The coping mechanism (regulator and cognator) act in relation to the adaptive modes.[62]
4. If energy is freed from inadequate coping attempts, then it can be utilized to promote healing and wellness.[63]
5. If the coping mechanism (regulator and cognator) is ineffective, then ineffective behaviors result:
   a. If the regulator system is ineffective, then physiological data (blood pressure, pulse, respiration, etc.) will reflect the degree of ineffectiveness.
   b. If cognator system is ineffective, then the degree of ineffectiveness will be reflected in the degree of the client's awareness of needs, ability to identify goals, ability to select means to goals, and the degree to which goals are attainable. (Implied)
6. If the behavior of the client has been clearly specified, then the nurse can write goals of expected outcomes mutually agreed upon by both nurse and client.[64]
7. Behaviors will tend to be adaptive if the client can keep securing adequate information about the environment, maintain satisfac-

tory internal conditions for action and for processing information, and maintain autonomy.[65]

8. The adaptation level varies with the pooled effect of focal, contextual, and residual stimuli or stressors.[66]
9. If the effort to overcome stress is not sufficient, the coping mechanisms will be activated to produce greater responses.[67]
10. The nurse makes judgments about the effectiveness of adaptive response behaviors based on a value hierarchy of goals to be achieved and on the long-term effects of these behaviors.[68]
11. For the regulator system:
    a. The degree of internal and external stimuli influences the degree of physiological response.
    b. The degree to which nerve pathways are intact influences neural output effectors.
    c. Chemical and neural inputs influence the responsiveness of the endocrine glands to harmonally influence target organs in a manner to maintain equilibrium.
    d. Responses of the body alter stimuli.
    e. The magnitude of stimuli may be so great that the adaptive systems cannot maintain the body's equilibrium.[69]
12. For the cognator system:
    a. The optimum amount and clarity of input stimuli influences the adequacy of the cognator system's functioning.
    b. Intact pathways and perceptual/information-processing apparatus influence the adequacy of cognator systems.
    c. The degree of accuracy of the cognator processes influences the effectiveness of psychomotor response choices.
    d. The psychomotor response choices will be activated through intact effectors.
    e. Effector activity produces responses at the adaptive level determined by the cognator system.
    f. The level of adaptive responses to stimuli alters the stimuli.[70]
13. The meaning of perception will influence the body response.[71]
14. The regulator and cognator systems are associated through the process of perception.[72]
15. If stimuli cause behavior, then stimuli must be changed to change behavior.[73]
16. The client is enabled to reestablish equilibrium to the degree the nurse can accurately assess, diagnose, and implement changes in stimuli. (Implicit)

These, then, are the fundamental ways in which Roy relates the four major concepts of nursing—that is, nurse, client, health, and environment. In turn, she has developed these basic relationship statements into a series of detailed propositions that appear to be an intermediate step toward the development of research hypotheses for specific client case analysis.[74] Indeed, several chapters of her book are devoted to the use of the theory to analyze client situations involving the four adaptive modes.[75] Thus in Roy's theory the human being requiring nursing services is viewed as a living system having an imbalance of the adaptive modes and the internal processor systems. The behavioral outputs are indicative of the degree of inadequate coping attempts, and are the source of data for the nurse to assess. In this nursing process, the nurse's goal is to promote effective functioning of the adaptive modes and the internal processor systems to achieve the highest level of wellness possible for the client.

Evaluation

The final step in our plan of theory analysis is to determine the value of the theory to nursing as a discipline and a practice profession. The criteria we have selected are those suggested in Chapter 11: parsimony, scope, applicability, generalizability, agreement with known data, relevant research, and importance to the discipline.

Parsimony. Economy of verbiage and the use of simple, clear statements are indicative of parsimony. Although Roy's theory is not presented succinctly in one publication, it is still a relatively simple theory having a small number of major concepts. In order to grasp it, however, we must consult about half a dozen references. The theory has apparently been developing over the course of a decade, and this has resulted in discrepancies between earlier and recent statements; this is also reported by Wagner.[76] In addition, numerous relationship statements have been developed; theories characterized by parsimony have a limited number of such statements. In order to make this theory more readily available to practicing nurses—and not just graduate students and nursing scholars—it seems a brief, simple statement of the total theory would be helpful in developing its research and application. It would also be helpful if throughout the statement one concept were used to refer to one phenomenon. For example, in Roy's writings the concepts "adaptive modes" and "internal processor system" are defined quite clearly and distinctly, but the phrase "the coping mechanism" is used in an ambiguous manner. Thus the reader is left wondering whether or not the coping mechanism refers to one or both, or to parts of both, of the adaptive modes and the internal processor system. However, the examples of the theory's application to client situations seem well separated from theoretical discussions, thus avoiding a confusing mix of theory and example. In summary, it appears that the theory could be stated a bit more succinctly. To do so would perhaps increase its availability and popularity among practicing nurses.

Scope. The amount of territory covered in this theory is very broad in that it is concerned with the total phenomena of the nurse assessing and providing care as it "happens" in client-nurse dyads in clinical practice. It excludes consideration of the nurse as a person and/or professional, except to implicitly picture the nurse as an intelligent, analytical, goal-directed professional who thoughtfully analyzes data, diagnoses, confers with the client, and takes nursing actions. The focus is on the individual client's coping behavior, particularly those aspects commonly associated with bio-physio-psycho-social perspectives of nursing care. While wholeness is emphasized, there seems to be some "conceptual slippage" or inconsistency between the bio-physio-psycho-social arrangement of the examples provided and the theoretical definition of the human being as a living system. This probably reflects the "real" world of nursing practice and its literature, which typically use the bio-physio-psycho-social set to define Man. To logically follow from the theoretical definitions, the adaptive modes and the internal processor systems of the living human systems need to be the organizing principle for the genre of theoretical examples. This is particularly true if we are to follow the eristic style of thinking, which Roy seems to do. However, the theory does provide an excellent framework, mapping out the extensive territory of nursing, as Brower and Baker testify.[77] They used Roy's theory in teaching and found it helpful in achieving mastery of the nurse practitioner role for graduate students.

Limitations. There are several limitations to Roy's theory. First, the fact that she borrows concepts from the theories of other disciplines without redefining those concepts in terms of specific nursing theory can pose problems both for the reader and ultimately for the researcher who attempts to operationalize them. For example, the terms "target tissue" and "reinforcement" seem to be drawn from stress-adaptation and behaviorist condition-response theories. Second, while the theory proposes to provide a "holistic" view of the client, the "whole person" does not seem to include the spiritual dimensions, the life force within. In other words, it seems to omit the humanistic and existential aspects of being human. However, the self-concept category provides space in which other theories speaking to these characteristics could reasonably be compatible with Roy's theory. As the theory now stands, it seems to imply that "Man" is defined only as a survival-oriented, behaviorist (condition-response), amoral, living system. Some nurses would feel the need to amplify this definition. Third, the theory's concepts have yet to be operationalized, and some plan of measurement needs to be developed so that extensive research programs can be undertaken. While Roy and her colleagues may have made advances that have yet to be published, the theory's concepts still seem, for the most part, to be at the ordinal or nominal levels. These factors are of particular relevance in limiting the scope of Roy's theory. It is anticipated that such limitations will be given due consideration and eliminated within the next decade.

Applicability. Roy's theory provides an excellent, broad theoretical perspective, and other theories can be used to supplement it. For example, a theory of the growth and development model may be helpful to use with Roy's adaptation theory in a pediatric or family-care clinical setting. By the same token, a theory of the symbolic interaction model can be used to enrich the nurse-client dialogue in the assessment and implementation of the nursing process. Roy's theory also seems potentially compatible with the medical models of pathophysiology and related theories, taxonomies, and so on. Its use has the potential to foster communication between physicians and nurses. The designer of this theory is a nurse and it is applicable to nursing because it has evolved out of Roy's own experiences in the field—that is, from what nursing practice *is*.

Generalizability and agreement with known data. In her writings, Roy presents numerous references to theory and research in other disciplines as well as nursing, and these provide a factual foundation for her own theory. This theory seems to have great potential generalizability, and it seems to agree with known data from the systems and stress-adaptation literature as well as from the nursing literature.

Relevant research. Extensive, relevant research has yet to be conducted to determine the validity of the theory, as has been noted by Roy herself.[78] Wagner also encountered some difficulty in determining into which adaptive mode a specific observed behavior belonged. Furthermore, the theory's use in intensive care areas required considerable revision of the nursing process tool she developed.[79] However, on the whole, the theory seems to be potentially applicable and generalizable to all areas of nursing practice, pending further study and research.

Importance to the discipline. Roy's nursing theory of adaptation is a significant contribution to the nursing knowledge base. It focuses on what nursing *is*, and this is an important requirement of nursing theories as identified by Ellis.[80] It provides a means of organizing most of nursing knowledge for curriculum development in nursing education. The nursing diagnosis is significantly advanced by this theory, which meets many current practice needs.[81] Use of an extensive data base obtained through the nurse's own assessment fosters prudent independence of thinking and acting for the clinical nurse. The theory also provides direction for the delineation of a common nursing role, distinguishing nursing from those health care providers who often seem to tread on our territory or vice versa.

SUMMARY

Roy's nursing theory seems to have the potential to meet all the functions of a theory: descriptive, explanatory, predictive, and prescriptive. Thus it may become the most favored theory in nursing . . . for a while. . . .

NOTES

1. Dorothy E. Johnson, "Development of Theory: A Requisite for Nursing as a Primary Health Profession," in Norma L. Chaska, ed., *The Nursing Profession: Views Through the Mist* (New York: McGraw-Hill, 1978), p. 213.
2. Sister Callista Roy and Sharon L. Roberts, *Theory Construction in Nursing: An Adaptation Model* (Englewood Cliffs, N.J.: Prentice-Hall, 1981).
3. Brent D. Ruben and John Y. Kim, eds., *General Systems Theory and Human Communication* (Rochelle Park, N.J.: Hayden, 1975), pp. 4–5.
4. Ervin Laszlo, "Basic Constructs of Systems Philosophy," Ruben and Kim, eds., *General Systems Theory and Human Communication*, p. 66.
5. Ruben and Kim, *General Systems Theory and Human Communication*, p. 4.
6. Ibid., pp. 1–2.
7. Ludwig von Bertalanffy, "General Systems Theory," in Ruben and Kim, *General Systems Theory and Human Communication*, pp. 6–9.
8. Ibid., p. 9.
9. Ibid., pp. 6–19.
10. David H. Smith, "Communication Research and the Idea of Process," *Speech Monographs* 39 (August 1972):174–182.
11. Ibid.
12. Leonard C. Hawes, "Elements of a Model for Communication Processes," *Quarterly Journal of Speech* 59 (February 1973):9.
13. Ervin Laszlo, "Basic Constructs of Systems Philosophy," in Ruben and Kim, eds., *General Systems Theory and Human Communication*, pp. 66–77.

14. Sister Callista Roy, "Decision-making by the Physically Ill and Adaptation During Illness" (Ph.D. diss., University of California, Los Angeles, 1971).

15. Sister Callista Roy, *Introduction to Nursing: An Adaptation Model* (Englewood Cliffs, N.J.: Prentice-Hall, 1976); Roy and Roberts, *Theory Construction in Nursing*; Sister Callista Roy, "Adaptation: A Conceptual Framework for Nursing," *Nursing Outlook* 18 (March 1970):42–45; and, Sister Callista Roy, "Adaptation: A Basis for Nursing Practice," *Nursing Outlook* 19 (April 1971):254–257.

16. Julia B. George, chairperson, *Nursing Theories: The Base for Professional Nursing Practice (A Report of the Nursing Theories Conference Group)* (Englewood Cliffs, N.J.: Prentice-Hall, 1980); Mija Kim and Derry Ann Moritz, eds., *Classification of Nursing Diagnosis: Proceedings of the Third and Fourth National Conferences* (New York: McGraw-Hill, 1982).

17. Sister Callista Roy, "The Roy Adaptation Modes: Comment," *Nursing Outlook* 24 (November 1976):690–691; Roy and Roberts, *Theory Construction in Nursing*, p. 42.

18. H. Helson. *Adaptation Level Theory: An Experimental and Systematic Approach to Behavior* (New York: Harper & Row, 1964).

19. Roy and Roberts, *Theory Construction in Nursing*, pp. 50, 53.

20. Ibid., pp. 51, 58.

21. Ibid., p. 52.

22. Ibid., p. 51.

23. Ibid.

24. Ibid., p. 52.

25. Ibid.

26. Ibid., pp. 53, 58.

27. Ibid., p. 53.

28. Ibid.

29. Ibid., p. 45.

30. Ibid., p. 36.

31. Ibid., p. 59.

32. Ibid., p. 44.

33. Ibid., p. 53.

34. Ibid., p. 59.

35. Ibid., p. 45.

36. Ibid., p. 49.

37. Ibid., pp. 36, 53, 81.

38. Ibid., p. 63.

39. Ibid., p. 44.

40. Ibid., p. 45.

41. Ibid., p. 47.

42. Ibid., p. 37.

43. Ibid., pp. 20–28.

44. Ibid., p. 31.

45. Ibid., p. 45.

46. Ibid., p. 55.
47. Ibid., p. 42.
48. Ibid., p. 43.
49. Ibid., pp. 43, 57.
50. Ibid., p. 60.
51. Ibid., p. 63.
52. Ibid., pp. 63, 285–286.
53. Ibid., p. 67.
54. Ibid., pp. 43–44.
55. Ibid., p. 285.
56. Ibid., p. 55.
57. Ibid., p. 67.
58. Ibid., pp. 44–46, 286–287.
59. Ibid., pp. 46–48.
60. Ibid., p. 46.
61. Ibid., p. 45.
62. Ibid., p. 43.
63. Ibid., p. 45.
64. Ibid., p. 47.
65. Ibid., p. 57.
66. Ibid., p. 59.
67. Ibid.
68. Ibid., p. 57.
69. Ibid., p. 62.
70. Ibid., p. 65.
71. Ibid., p. 67.
72. Ibid.
73. Ibid., p. 287.
74. Ibid., pp. 62, 65.
75. Ibid., pp. 72–283.
76. Patricia Wagner, "The Roy Adaptation Model: Testing the Adaptation Model in Practice," *Nursing Outlook* 24 (November 1976):682.
77. H. Terri Francis Brower and Bryie Jo Baker, "The Roy Adaptation Model: Using the Adaptation Model in a Practitioner Curriculum," *Nursing Outlook* 24 (November 1976):686–689.
78. Roy and Roberts, *Theory Construction in Nursing*, pp. 289–290.
79. Wagner, "The Roy Adaptation Model," p. 257.
80. Rosemary Ellis, "Characteristics of Significant Theories," in Margaret E. Hardy, ed. *Theoretical Foundations for Nursing* (New York: MSS Information, 1973), p. 89.
81. Sister Callista Roy, "A Diagnostic Classification System for Nursing," *Nursing Outlook* 23 (February 1975):90–94.

FOUR

Building a Theory: Humanistic Nursing Communication

A theory is a set of interrelated constructs (concepts), definitions and propositions that present a systematic view of phenomena by specifying relations among variables, with the purpose of explaining and predicting the phenomena.[1]

We have used Kerlinger's definition of a theory as a basis for our theory analysis and have identified four major elements—assumptions, concepts, relationship statements, and evaluation—that are essential to all theories. The identification of these elements has been shown to be a means of analyzing any theory. Ultimately, as their familiarity with a number of theories increases, nurses will be able to approach the clinical practice of nursing with many theoretical perspectives and increase the predictability of their nursing practice outcomes.

Of course, individual nurses usually have their own personal theories of nursing. Generally these philosophies, perspectives, or speculations concern the values and realities of nursing activities. Some nurses may wish to build their own formal theories, but they shy away from this because the theory-building process is not widely known or discussed in their field. However, in recent years the topic of theories, theory analysis, and even theory-building has increasingly been found on the agendas of workshops and educational programs. And in the next few years, we believe that discussions of theory will be much more common. Thus professional nurses will need and want to know how to build a theory, even if it is only a brief statement of their own personal philosophy of nursing. Indeed, within the next decade, we predict that the application of nursing theories will be an expected part of clinical nursing and will be included in criteria to be met for the accreditation of hospitals and similar health agencies. As a part of this process, nurses will be expected to know about many nursing theories.

In this final part of our book, we will present a new theory of nursing, that of humanistic nursing communication, attempting to describe how each of its four major elements were developed, as well as present the theory in its totality. This theory has been developed over a five-year period, and portions of it have already been presented in an earlier work. You may wish to consult this source for an in-depth understanding of the research behind the theory.[2]

The steps in theory-building correspond exactly to the four elements we have used to analyze a theory: (1) identifying assumptions; (2) defining categories of phenomena (that is, concepts), (3) establishing relationships between or among these categories or concepts, and (4) evaluating them for practical value. However, although this is the logical sequence, it is not necessarily the sequence in which a theory develops.

In building a theory, thoughts can occur quite randomly. Thus the theorist needs to establish goals, deliberately assign time for thinking, and keep jotting down ideas. In this process, the mind naturally seeks a hierarchy or structure of ideas, and soon a logical sequence emerges. This was true of the theory of humanistic nursing communication, even though, for our purposes, it must be presented sequentially according to the four steps or elements outlined above.

Theories that are designated specifically as nursing theories concern the concepts of human beings as "clients" experiencing "health" needs in an "environment" or situation in which "nursing" care is provided by a "nurse." Such concepts must be present in order for a theory to be classified as a nursing theory. In presenting these concepts, the theory of humanistic nursing communication uses the symbolic interactionist model, which is described in the following section.

THE SYMBOLIC INTERACTIONIST MODEL

In searching for ways to overcome concerns about the meaninglessness of life experiences, and in seeking ways to make day-to-day experiences more meaningful, a group of theorists and scholars concluded that human beings create meaning out of everyday experiences through collaboration within personal relationships. Thus they assume that the study of communication between people—that is, interpersonal communication—can provide knowledge and understanding of how "humanization" occurs and how this development of meaningfulness through collaboration is achieved.

The study of human communication is, however, one of the most complex tasks undertaken by mankind.[3] As Smith and Williamson, remind us: "The concept of meaning—possibly the most advanced achievement of animals on the earth—has been reached only by man and perhaps the dolphin."[4] They also suggest that interpersonal communication may not have been examined closely in the past because it seems, at least on the surface, so simple, so ordinary—as if it were too obvious to be important.[5] Thus it has only been in our own century that theorists and scholars have focused much attention on the study of communication between people. In the course of this, numerous communication models have been developed: psychoanalysis, information theory and cybernetics, transactional analysis, and symbolic interaction. The humanistic nursing communication theory is based on the latter.

In this section, the assumptions of the symblic interactionist model will be discussed in regard to its description of Man, the purposes of communication, the use of language, motivation, and its chief integrating concept, the "self." And since the models used in a discipline influence the characteristics of its knowledge base, we will also include some speculations about how the symbolic interactionist model can influence the knowledge base of nursing.

Symbolic interactionists as a group tend to describe Man rather explicitly. For example, Kenneth Burke describes Man as a symbol-using, misusing animal, inventor of the negative (no, nonexistence, rules, laws, and so on), seeking a hierarchy within society (practicing one-upmanship among one another), separated from his natural condition by instruments of his own making (because of the ability to symbolize and use language), and goaded by perfection (aware of how things *should* be, but never quite able to attain such a state).[6] In Burke's view, Man is both action (animalistic) and motion (humanistic) in that he shares with animals the constraints of physical reality, time, and space (having the use of only five senses and being restricted to a particular slice of time and space). However, because of his ability to symbolize, he is lifted out of this restricted interaction of time and space. Man is able to move via thought into the past and the future, and he is able to think of things that are not present, nonexistent, and abstract in addition to thinking of things that are present and have objective referents.[7]

Theorists and scholars who can be labeled symbolic interactionists include Burke, Buber, Mead, Duncan, Langer, Casserier, Cooley, Dewey, and Sullivan. All of these individuals seem to have developed their ideas out of a dissatisfaction with the linear, speaker-centered, narrow, and traditional communication theory that existed in the early 1900s. And they all had the opportunity to study theories of many disciplines, particularly those of European and American psychology, sociology, and social psychology.[8]

The objective of communication for the symbolic interactionists is primarily to find meaning and understanding. Burke, for example, states that communication exists to unite Men. He sees Man as being continually divided by hierarchies and going through a series of interlocking moments in which agreements are broken and adjustments are consequently necessary. In his view, communication is the means whereby Man achieves "consubstantiality"—elements or levels of this include sympathizing, categorizing, and identifying, which is the highest level of unity. Through the use of symbolism, Burke sees Man as being able to select increasingly more ambiguous words in order to transcend a level of conflict and become joined in some cooperative effort of mutual concern. Although Buber is usually classified as an existentialist, he is also often considered a symbolic interactionist. In his communication theory, the "I-Thou" relationship is a communication which, though transitory, is timeless in nature, and it focuses upon the commitment to an intense relationship with another person. In this "I-Thou" relationship, the individual seeks to capture a bit of heaven on earth by trying to relate to the element of God that is assumed to be in all humans—that is, the individual tries to reach God through human communing. This relationship is contrasted with the "I-It" relationship, which consists of an "I" looking at another person or thing as an "it," and using that "it" within a specific slice of time and space. Buber states that examples of this can be found in business and economic relationships. In such relationships there is no commitment; rather, there are only directives. The "it" is merely an instrument for the use of the "I."[9]

For the symbolic interactionists, language is used by human beings to reveal reality. Thus, for Buber, language is the means whereby the individual can achieve the "I-Thou" relationship, and reality is not important. Perhaps a more typical symbolic interactionist view of language is that of Burke, for whom language is the means whereby human beings label reality. Burke explains this through the concept of a "terministic" screen (as seen in Figure 17) of past experiences, personality, and the total essence of the individual, which "selects, deflects, and reflects" reality in such a manner that reality is seen as if through a "fog of symbols." According to Burke, reality probably exists "out there," but we can never know it directly.[10]

For the symbolic interactionist, communication motivates humans,

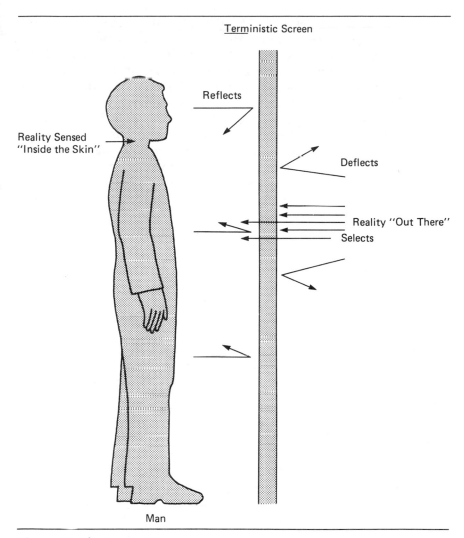

Figure 17. The terministic screen.

and motivation is symbolic in nature. Thus Buber places motivation in the "I-It" relationship; the "I" is motivated to use the other, who is perceived as an "it." Burke proposes that human motivation lies in our words themselves. For example, the words "to do one's duty" are motivating in that the individual tends to be moved to perform whatever activity or behavior is implied with the situation. Burke also sees motivation as lying beyond symbolization. In his view, we use symbols to pull motivation into our awareness and thus label it. Using the concept of motivation, Burke describes a means of analyzing communicative situations. To do so, he devised a tool, the "dramatistic pentad," as the calculus of motives. This consists of a set of elements to be considered in analyzing a communicative situation: the agent, the agency, the scene, the purpose (motive), and the act.[11] The function of the pentad is to reveal the total motivation, which would ordinarily remain hidden. An example of pentad analysis is provided by Fisher in the analysis of the motivation of a man named Blank White, who committed murder and suicide. Here the problems of guilt, resulting victimage, and mortification ,are revealed in a most interesting manner. In short, Fisher proves that the pentad is effective.[12]

For the symbolic interactionist, meaning resides within and between people, and the primary integrating factors are the "self" or "self-system" and the "role." Thus it is through interpersonal communication and social interaction that the self is developed and sustained. As Smith and Williamson explain it:

> Those theorists observed that human infants are born not with a developed language, but with a capacity to learn human languages. Infants do not speak English or Chinese when they emerge from the womb; they learn the language of the group in which they are reared. . . . With experience the child begins to internalize certain roles which eventually come together to form what the child finally experiences as the self. With the further development of language, the child begins to understand how other "selves" would react in situations similar to the child's experiences. Finally, each child develops the ability to empathize with others in situations that he or she has not experienced.[13]

It is clear, then, that symbolic interaction focuses on the social aspects of human communication. And here the concept of "role" provides a dual perspective. The sociological role refers to an established set of behaviors prescribed by society for particular roles, such as the mother, father, teacher, lawyer, and so on. The psychological role refers to the attitude with which an individual fulfills the sociological role. Thus the sociological role of the nurse may be fulfilled by assuming either a caring or a careless attitude. We can see from this that the concepts of self and role provide central foci for the study of interpersonal communication, of the development and maintenance of self-concepts, and of the determination of meaningfulness in human existence.[14]

For human beings, meaning arises out of relationships with others—that is, from communing. This involves a unifying, or a joining together, of two or more people so that their individuality is lost and a new unit is formed. They become a dyad, a triad, and so on. In the same instant, however, individual differences are retained so that the relationship is unique and special. Thus meaningful communication is more than a mere transfer of information, as from a computer disk to a printer. Instead, meaning requires that the behavior of one person be perceived by another, that one person experience another. And while such experience is a very private matter, there is at the same time a *shared* experience of reality among human beings—shared through symbols or language. A significant part of this shared experience includes either loneliness, alienation, and dehumanization or intimacy, unity, and humanization.

The choice of the symbolic interaction model has far-reaching effects upon the developing knowledge base of nursing since it studies communication phenomena as a dynamic relationship in which both speaker and receiver are the equal elements, as opposed to the traditional speaker-oriented or receiver-oriented perspectives. An example of this can be seen in the hospice context, in which nurses communicate carefully, listening for feelings, concerns, and hopes that are expressed by fatally ill clients. Similar phenomena can be observed in the nurse-client communication that takes place in specialty or intensive-care contexts, such as renal dialysis centers and rape crisis centers. In the administration of nursing services, many health organizations are seeking greater individual involvement in communication systems through the decentralization of the organization. In addition, the symbolic interactionist model has the potential to provide a more holistic view of the human being. The holistic perspective encompasses the total person rather than just a disease or a symptom. In it, equilibrium of body, mind, spirit, and environment is emphasized, and the person is seen as being primarily responsible for the changing that must take place.[16] This model will perhaps provide a more accurate view of nursing communication than any other.

The questions that are asked by disciplines using the symbolic interactionist model can be summarized by returning to Burke's pentad. The "agent" is the speaker and/or receiver. What kind of person is this? The "agency" is the instrument or line of thought—the words, the attitudes, and other expressive modes a person uses in communicating. Why has this person chosen to communicate in this way? The "scene" includes all factors related to the background of the communication—the context, the environment, and the relationship. What factors of the scene have significant influences upon the totality of experiencing another? The "purpose" focuses upon the motives of each person. To what degree is the speaker sincere or deceptive, and why is this communication occurring? Finally, the "act" asks what happened or what has transpired. In summary, Burke states that the process involves: "what was done (act), when or where it was done (scene), who did it (agent), how he did it (agency), and why (purpose)."[17] Such questions focus not only on the bio-physical-psycho-social but also on the metaphysical phenomena of human experience.

Research within the symbolic interactionist model will tend to be process oriented, eventually giving attention to multiple variables within one study. The use of subjective data, field studies, interviewers, observers, and audiovisual recording of data are only a few of the approaches that are possible and appropriate in the study of communicative interactions in nursing practice. Because research with this model will tend to be less restrictive than that of some of the more formal, classical designs, it is highly possible that new and unique approaches to the study of communication in nursing will emerge with its use. With the symbolic interactionist model, the goals of nursing practice will focus on achieving unity, congruence, and agreement—and perhaps even intimacy—in nurse/client relationships. Thus the symbolic interactionist model seems to offer considerable support to the heart of nursing, which is the interpersonal relationship between the nurse and the client.

THE THEORIST

The author of the theory of humanistic nursing communication is Bonnie Weaver Duldt, a scholar who has spent most of her career in the field of nursing education. Acutely aware of the numerous dehumanizing and alienating aspects of nurses' experience, Duldt frequently observed formerly bright, enthusiastic students of nursing becoming disillusioned and disheartened graduates who seemed to stop trying to maintain ideals of quality nursing care. In addition, she also observed that communications with health-care providers seemed to be the central issue of complaints that were voiced by many of the recipients of that care. After focusing in her doctoral dissertation on the angry messages nurses receive from others, Duldt identified the anger-dismay syndrome in a later research effort.

Duldt sees the future context of health-care delivery becoming a more complex and difficult one. Thus she proposes that nurses' perspectives be changed because it is unlikely that the context will change. She believes nurses can be helped to cope with dehumanization and be made aware of the range of communicative choices that are available to them. Ultimately, in her view, nurses can be helped to feel better about themselves, and clients, in turn, can feel better about their care. This can be achieved through the study of humanizing, meaningful interpersonal communications.

In line with this goal, Duldt has expanded her research to include other alienating communications such as verbal abuse and sexual harassment, while giving continued consideration to describing and defining humanizing, unifying, and meaningful communications. Her theory of humanistic nursing communication has evolved to its present state since Duldt completed her doctoral work at the University of Kansas (1978) in speech communication and human relations, majoring in small task-group communication and minoring in organizational communication.

Unlike Roy, Duldt does not refer to herself as a theorist but as a practicing nurse educator. And her theory itself may indeed provide a helpful and practical framework for teaching communication in academic and service educational settings. In this context, the way the theory is presented is perhaps as important as the theory itself.

Because she is concerned about the gap between theory and practice, Duldt hopes that her manner (or a similar one) of writing and analyzing theories can be developed so that a greater portion of the nursing population will also find the abstract, theoretical side of nursing attractive. Just as computer scientists are seeking to write "user-friendly" computer software, so nurse theorists, scholars, and educators need to seek succinct ways of writing "nurse-friendly" theories. The significance of this contribution to nursing will be determined primarily by you, our readers, since Duldt's theory has not been formally tested, other than in her own research efforts.

Although the humanistic communication theory has been shared with many groups of nurses through courses, workshops, seminars, and lectures, its first formal statement is being presented in this book. The theory and research that serve as its basis have been presented in an earlier publication; the elements of humanizing and dehumanizing communication have also been defined extensively and reported in this same publication.[18] The application of the humanistic nursing communication theory and Situational Leadership theory to nursing leadership contexts will be the focus of Duldt's third text, coauthored with Paul Hersey.[19] Like Roy, her work has only begun.

NOTES

1. Fred N. Kerlinger, *Foundations of Behavioral Research*, 2nd ed. (New York: Holt, Rinehart and Winston, 1973), p. 9.
2. Bonnie Weaver Duldt, Kim Giffin, and Bobby R. Patton, *Interpersonal Communication in Nursing* (Philadelphia: F. A. Davis, 1983).
3. Dennis R. Smith and L. Keith Williamson, *Interpersonal Communication: Roles, Rules, Strategies, and Games* (Dubuque, Ia.: Wm. C. Brown, 1977), p. 5.

4. Ibid., p. 6.

5. Ibid.

6. Kenneth Burke, *Language as Symbolic Action: Essays on Life, Literature, and Method* (Berkeley: University of California Press, 1966), pp. 1–16.

7. Ibid., pp. 3–24.

8. Smith and Williamson, *Interpersonal Communication*, pp. 9–27.

9. Burke, *Language as Symbolic Action*; Martin Buber, *I and Thou*, trans. by Walter Kaufmann (New York: Scribner's, 1970).

10. Burke, *Language as Symbolic Action*.

11. In a conversation during a visit to the University of Kansas campus in 1976, Dr. Burke later stated that "attitude" and "scope" should have been added to the set.

12. Jeanne Y. Fisher, "A Burkean Analysis of the Rhetorical Dimensions of a Multiple Murder and Suicide," *Quarterly Journal of Speech* 60 (April 1974):175–189.

13. Smith and Williams, *Interpersonal Communication*, p. 13.

14. Ibid., pp. 12–15.

15. Ibid., pp. 40–43; David K. Berlo, *The Process of Communication* (San Francisco: Rinehart, 1960), pp. 124–129; Jerome G. Manis and Bernard N. Meltzer, eds., *Symbolic Interaction: A Reader in Social Psychology* (Boston: Allyn and Bacon, 1967).

16. Patricia Anne Flynn, *Holistic Health: The Art and Science of Care* (Bowie, Md.: Robert J. Brady, 1980), pp. 12–13.

17. Kenneth Burke, *A Grammar of Motives* (Berkeley: University of California Press, 1969), pp. xv–xxiii.

18. Duldt, Giffin, and Patton, *Interpersonal Communication in Nursing*.

19. Bonnie W. Duldt and Paul Hersey, *Situational Leadership in Humanistic Nursing* (Englewood Cliffs, N.J.: Prentice-Hall, in press).

Assumptions

13

An assumption has been defined as a given, an assertion that is not tested. Thus assumptions provide a theory with a framework that does not move or change. These assumptions can be identified by the verbs a theory uses, verbs of the present tense that are descriptive.

In this chapter we will present a series of assertions that, taken together, represent the assumptions of Duldt's humanistic nursing communication theory. But where does a person get a set of assumptions? In Chapter 7, we identified a set of four elements that are involved in the process of developing assumptions: observing, remembering, analoguing, and expressing. While the development of a set of elements may seem easier than writing a set of assumptions, the main difference seems to us to be the amount of time and thought involved. Thus we will describe a "behind the author's eyes" view of how Duldt developed her assumptions, using observing, remembering, analoguing, and expressing as our organizing principles.

OBSERVING

The phenomena that is of interest to nurses is nursing itself, particularly the practice of nursing as it applies to each individual. Here, then, we have the basic criterion of a nursing theory: it must concern something that is happening that involves a nurse and a client (a human being), the client's health, and the client's environment.[1] However, thinking about a nurse, a client, health, and the environment is probably too much for most students of nursing theory, particularly at first. Consequently, we suggest that you select an area or aspect of nursing practice, and focus on that. For example, you could look at the skills performance of nurses and their clients' physical response. Or you could look at care plans for a group of clients having something in common, such as a mobility or oxygenation problem. Just be sure to limit the theory to the areas of nursing that are most familiar to you. Then look at theories that have been developed and take note of what has been omitted from them. What are you doing in your own practice that no theorist has yet taken into consideration? When considering this question, include conversations with others and readings of others' works in your observations. Listen to your own feelings and, above all, trust your own intuition and judgment about what is important.

In proceeding as outlined above, Duldt chose to look at the interpersonal communication occurring between a nurse, clients, and the nurse's colleagues and coworkers. However, from this area of concern she excluded therapeutic communications, which constitute a specialized way of interacting with a particular category of client, the psychiatric patient. She did this because there are already numerous theories about how to communicate with this group of patients, and also because there are few theories that seek to help nurses communicate with "normal" or "regular" people.[2]

It was evident to Duldt that most people who seek health care are "regular" people who tend to be quite capable of coping with life's problems, even with illness and death. In addition, she noted that many of these people seem to think that doctors and nurses communicate in an abnormal manner. To them, they seem condescending, distant, and secretive. Consequently, doctors and nurses are not always viewed by patients as a helpful resource, and needed care is sometimes bypassed or ignored by the very people nurses are seeking to help. Based on these observations, it seemed to Duldt that a broadly based communication theory was needed in order to help nursing become an attractive and trustworthy resource to more people who have health problems.

Yet Duldt also noted another need. While many nurses cooperate and maintain effective working relationships with their colleagues, at the same time there seem to be too many nurses who are uncooperative, rude, and irritable. New graduates of nursing schools continually complain about the lack of support and the limited efforts that are made to include the novice in the work group. Even the seasoned, experienced nurse who tries to take on a new administrative position can be faced with malicious behavior and resentment on the part of other nurses. Staff nurses can experience anger and dismay, as well as emotional distress, due to angry physicians who verbally abuse and sexually harass them.[3] And supervisors often seem unnecessarily harsh, almost verbally punishing, in response to routine errors or equipment failures, which often are not the fault of the nurse involved.

Clearly there is an urgent need to correct these negative attitudes and unattractive patterns of interaction. Thus Duldt believes that a theory is needed that can look at the unpleasant as well as the pleasant communicative realities as experienced by nurses at all levels, but particularly by those at the staff nurse level. After all, it is the staff nurse who receives the greatest amount of negative or dehumanizing communications, and is therefore most in need of a theory that would help identify negative attitudes and provide means of coping with destructive or dehumanizing interaction patterns used by peers, co-workers, and colleagues.

One major problem in the communication between a nurse and peers or colleagues is the nurse's lack of power and the reluctance of superiors to use their power. Consider, for example, the situation in which one nurse asked another nurse to help in the delivery room by taking over the care of the newborn. The other nurse just stood there and made no move to help, for no apparent reason. So the first nurse proceeded to provide all the necessary care herself. She discussed this at length in a workshop on anger, revealing how angry and helpless she felt. Other staff nurses from the same hospital reported similar experiences with this same nurse. But the supervisors and head nurses, it seems, had been reluctant to write up the uncooperative behavior, confront the nurse, demand that she change, and, if she did not change, move to have her fired. Because peers have a choice in accepting or rejecting another's efforts to influence them, inappropriate choices need to be handled by supervisors in order to maintain the focus of attention on the client rather than on any interpersonal undercurrents that may exist among staff members.

These are some of the observations that Duldt made in viewing the phenomena of communication that nurses experience. Of all these observations, certain ones were remembered.

REMEMBERING

Those phenomena that are remembered are often those that are not explained, those that may be disturbing, and those that remain unresolved. For example, many of the communications experienced by nurses seem unpleasant at best, yet the essence of nursing itself is seen by the consumer, by the prospective nursing student, and by graduate nurses alike as being just the reverse. Thus the nurse is seen as the lady with the soft step, the gentle touch, and the lighted candle. To be a nurse is to help others, a goal that to many is the ultimate purpose of life. Why, then, is the nurse seemingly the target of so many unpleasant messages from others? Why does the nurse seemingly behave so curtly to clients? And why do so many nurses leave the field after expending so much time, money, and effort on their education and credentials. These are all questions for which Duldt attempted to find answers.

ANALOGUING

We have suggested earlier that analogies and metaphors often are helpful in explaining new phenomena because they allow us to borrow from the familiar to find similarities and differences in new areas of knowledge. This is basically what Duldt was able to do.

First, she thought of communication as being in two categories, attractive and unattractive. These were later termed "humanizing" and "dehumanizing." The difficulty with categories, however, is that all data must fit into either one or the other. But in the communication that others reported, and that Duldt herself experienced, there seemed to be gradations of each—and sometimes just a certain neutrality of feelings. Thus it seemed that there might be a continuum of attitudes, extending from humanizing through neutrality to dehumanizing, much like the yin and yang forces of the Chinese philosophy of Taoism.[4]

For pragmatic reasons, the continuum was chosen because it is more readily adapted to statistics and the flow of Western thought. Thus a determination was made: in the judgment of the theorist, the analogy of choice to be used in this case was that believed to be most readily understood by members of the discipline and profession of nursing. This choice will tend to stimulate more research because it will fit commonly used statistical tools. Based on this choice, the theorist must next express the assumptions that have been identified.

EXPRESSING

The expression of assumptions is usually vocal at first, but they can be written down as soon as the theorist's thoughts seem to settle into a consistent pattern. This usually does not occur quickly, and it often involves several steps not necessarily in sequence. A first step is for the theorist simply to write out statements of assumptions quickly, with little editing, and set them aside for a few days. Periodic review and revision of these statements allows the theorist ample time for thought, as well as for careful editing as assumptions become clearer. During this process, the theorist often becomes aware of assumptions that have been omitted, or assumptions that are really unnecessary and can be deleted.

A second step involves discussing the assumptions with others and asking questions about others' beliefs and perceptions. Such discussions are often a source of new ideas or opposing views. Through them, the theorist learns to develop arguments that support certain assumptions and defend them against opposing views. Sometimes it is helpful to include people other than nurses in such discussions. After all, philosophers, members of the clergy, physicians, historians, and members of other disciplines can be very helpful in presenting perspectives that, while specific to their own area, still have a bearing on events and phenomena in nursing.

Generally, the broader the influence derived from other disciplines in the process of stating assumptions, the more reliable and valid the theory tends to be. Accordingly, Duldt went through the steps identified above and became influenced by three major disciplines—philosophy, speech communication, and nursing. In the paragraphs that follow, her assumptions are presented according to their relation to these three disciplines.

The following assumptions are derived from a study of philosophy, particularly humanistic and existential thought:

1. Human beings exist in a "here and now" existential context from which there is no escape.
2. Human beings are continually concerned with such existential elements as: being, becoming, choice, freedom, responsibility, solitude, loneliness, pain, struggle, tragedy, meaning, dread, uncertainty, despair, and death.
3. All elements of existential beings and the communication imperative are salient issues to be dealt with in critical life situations.
4. Growth and change arise from within the individual and to a considerable degree depend upon one's choice.
5. The nurse shares with the client all characteristics of being human.

Those assumptions that reflect the influence of communication theory and research are:

6. Survival is based on one's ability to communicate with others in order to share feelings and facts about the environment and ways of coping.
7. The environment is a "booming, buzzing" world of strange sensations that must be sorted out in order to determine which are most important; this sorting is achieved through communication with other people.
8. The need to communicate is an innate imperative for human beings.
9. Due to innate fallacies, human beings use and misuse all capabilities, especially the ability to communicate.
10. The way in which a person communicates determines what that person becomes.

11. Interpersonal communication is a humanizing factor that is an innate element of the nursing process (assessment, planning, implementation, and evaluation) and of the communication that occurs between nurses and clients, nurses and peers, and nurses and professional colleagues.
12. Evaluation of a person's own communication skills is subjective; each individual must make his or her own social decisions and choices about communication behavior and choose to change, depending upon his or her ability to utilize feedback.

Finally, the following assumptions are derived from nursing:

13. The purpose of nursing is to intervene to support, maintain, and augment the client's state of health.
14. A human being functions as a unique, whole system responding openly to the environment.

In addition to deriving assumptions from particular areas of study, the theorist ultimately is able to state assumptions that seem to be uniquely synthesized and specific to the particular theory that is being developed. The following assumptions that Duldt makes seem to fit this description:

15. Health, satisfaction, and success in a person's life and work—in other words, that person's state of being—is derived from feeling human.
16. Due to the bureaucratic and complex nature of the present health-care delivery systems, there is a tendency for clients and professionals to be treated in a dehumanizing manner and to relate to one another in a dehumanizing manner.
17. Humanizing patterns of communication can be learned and can enhance the nurse's awareness of and sensitivity to the client's state of being and of becoming.
18. The goal of the humanistic nurse is to break the communication cycle of dehumanizing attitudes and interaction patterns, replacing these with attitudes and patterns that humanize.
19. Interpersonal communication is the means by which the nurse becomes increasingly sensitive to and aware of the client's state of being, of the dynamic relationship between the client and his or her environment, and of the client's potential.

These, then, are the statements of assumption upon which Duldt's theory of humanistic nursing communication is based. These statements are assumed to be true without further testing.

We now have a description of the framework within which the concepts of the theory exist. The next task, to define the concepts of this theory, will be accomplished in the next chapter.

NOTES

1. Margaret Newman, *Theory Development in Nursing* (Philadelphia: F. A. Davis, 1979), p. 2; Margaret Newman, "Theory Development in Nursing: Where Has It Been and Where Is It Going?" Notes from a workshop sponsored by the Louisiana State University Medical Center School of Nursing, New Orleans, Louisiana, March 23, 1981.
2. Paul Hersey and Kenneth Blanchard, *Management of Organizational Behavior: Utilizing Human Resources*, 4th ed. (Englewood Cliffs, N.J.: Prentice-Hall, 1982).
3. Bonnie Weaver Duldt, "Helping Nurses Cope with the Anger-Dismay Syndrome," *Nursing Outlook* 30 (March 1982):168–174; Bonnie Weaver Duldt, "Sexual Harassment in Nursing," *Nursing Outlook* 30 (June 1982):336–343; Bonnie Weaver Duldt, Kim Giffin, and Bobby R. Patton, *Interpersonal Communication in Nursing* (Philadelphia: F. A. Davis, 1983), pp. 230–241.
4. Patricia Anne Randolph Flynn, *Holistic Health: The Art and Science of Care* (Bowie, Md.: Robert J. Brady, 1980), pp. 14–17.

Concepts

14

In Chapter 8, we defined concepts as labels that are applied to phenomena. Concepts are a "leap of faith" between a label or a group of utterances and some event, experience, or happening that human beings are aware of. In this chapter, we shall present the concepts that Duldt uses in her theory of humanistic nursing communication. These concepts include: "human being" (nurse, client, peer, and colleague); "critical life situation"; "health"; "environment"; "nursing"; and "communication."

In this chapter, we will describe the process Duldt used in developing definitions of these concepts, tracing the influence of the disciplines of philosophy, communication, and nursing. We will also present the complete definitions.

HUMAN BEING

The defining of the term "human being" is central to the theory of humanistic nursing communication. In defining the human being or Man, meaning both male and female, the influences of three disciplines need to be taken into consideration. Thus a human being needs to be defined as an existential and humanistic being, as a communicator, and as a client seeking nursing care. In the discussions that follow, we will present the reasoning behind the definition that was ultimately selected, showing the influence of the three disciplines. Then we will present the definition as it ultimately evolved.

In reviewing definitions of "human being" in the field of nursing, Duldt found that they did not fully denote those aspects of Man that she considered essential to a theory of humanistic nursing communication. She also found that nursing has borrowed many definitions from other disciplines, such as biology, psychology, and sociology—the bio-physical-psycho-social Man.

Biology is the science of living organisms. Thus biologists define the "human being" as a unique living creature and place *homo sapiens* in a taxonomy of all living creatures. They are concerned with how any living body works, and so they divide it into systems: circulatory, respiratory, urinary, and so on. In contrast, since psychology is the science of mind and behavior, members of this discipline focus on the "human being" as an individual who is behaving, interacting, thinking, and emoting. Thus they classify human beings as normal, neurotic, psychotic, depressed, and so on. However, animals rather than human subjects are used in many of their experiments and the results are generalized to apply to humans. Finally, sociology is the science of social institutions and relationships. It is therefore concerned with human beings living in groups, classifying such groups according to size, function, and so on.

In the dictionary, each of these disciplines is defined as a field of study having a particular territory of human knowledge. But if you look up nursing in the dictionary you will find that "nurse" means nourish at the breast, or a person who is skilled or trained in caring for the sick or infirm, especially under the supervision of a physician. In other words, nursing is defined as the profession of a nurse, the duties of a nurse. Dictionaries are society's storehouse of current word usage, and this is how nursing is defined by our society. It is not yet seen as a discipline. Consequently, we now have an additional expectation in terms of our definition of the client, the human being or Man. This definition now needs to define the entire field of nursing as a particular territory of human knowledge and skill specific to our discipline.

At this point, you may wonder why we should bother. What would be wrong with defining "human being" simply as a bio-physical-psycho-social entity? There are a number of reasons. First, these four divisions fail to adequately represent a human being as seen by a nurse. This is because three elements of the set relate to what goes on "inside the skin," and one to interactions among humans. Thus there is a central theme lacking in this set of elements. Furthermore, for those who would support the "wholeness" of Man, such a set is incomplete. Why not, for example, add a bit from other disciplines, such as law, ethics, religion, history, and so on?

We would not recommend defining Man according to Maslow's hierarchy of needs because those needs arise out of Man's interactions with the environment.[1] Some needs are not uniquely inherent in Man, but are shared with all life forms, for example, physiological and safety. For the same reason, we would also not recommend defining Man according to reactions to stress. After all, adaptation is also a process that is common to all life forms.[2]

As Burke reminds us, "a definition so sums things up that all properties attributed to the thing can be derived from the definition."[3] Thus we need to define Man according to unique, innate human characteristics that we can demonstrate are uniquely relevant to nursing as a discipline and a profession. We need a definition of "human being" that can serve as a classification or taxonomy for nursing as a discipline and a profession.

Over the centuries, human beings have been described by writers according to innate properties of humanness. One such definition is that of Kenneth Burke, a contemporary rhetorical and literary critic, philosopher, author, and communication theorist. In a brief essay, he defines Man as being something more than a psychological, social, political, or even cultural animal:

Man is
the symbol-using (symbol-making, symbol-misusing)
    animal,
inventor of the negative (or moralized by the negative),
separated from his natural condition by instruments of his
    own making,
goaded by the spirit of hierarchy (or moved by the sense of
    order),
and rotten with perfection.[4]

Each of these five phrases will now be reviewed in order to describe briefly Burke's meanings and to relate them to nursing.

In writing on Man as a symbol-using animal, Burke develops a comparison with birds. One day he entered his classroom to find all the windows and blinds up and a bird flying about the room. He describes what happened:

The windows were high, they extended almost to the ceiling; yet the bird kept trying to escape by batting against the ceiling rather than dipping down and flying out one of the open windows. . . . This particular bird's instinct was to escape by flying up . . . hence it ignored the easy exit through the windows. But how different things would be if the bird could speak and we could speak his language. What a simple statement would have served to solve his problem. "Fly down just a foot or so, and out one of the windows."[5]

However, Burke cites other examples of situations in which nonsymbolizing animals do behave in innovative ways; but because there is no way of communicating or recording any acts of genius for other members of the species to know and remember, no advancement is made. On the other hand, birds and other species are not susceptible to the misuse of symbols, as we are. Burke notes that only Man, the symbol-user, can be filled with hatred for people who are known only by hearsay, and that only Man can experience dread because of his expectations, most of which seldom occur. Indeed, much of Man's reality is based on symbols. As Burke puts it, "Take away our books and what little do we know about history, biography, even something so 'down to earth' as the relative position of seas and continents?"[6]

According to Burke, language is a set of labels or signs that we use like a road map to find our way about. Language changes our behavior because it is motivation; we live up to labels like "trustworthy," "patriotic," or even "foolish" and "dull." In relating this characteristic of Man to nursing, the very process of nursing is based on symbolism. For example, in assessment, we observe, label, and record. Because we can symbolize, we are able to build upon the learning, perceptions, and logic of both our predecessors and our contemporaries through the written and spoken use of language. Using symbols enables us to think abstractly, to use logic, to solve problems, and to learn. It also enables us to communicate perceptions regarding phenomena we have observed in our physical environment, in ourselves, in clients, and in relationships with others, and to communicate the feelings that arise from these perceptions. Many of our nursing interventions directly focus on helping our clients to communicate, as in the cases of the aphasic stroke victim, the retarded child, the emotionally disturbed, the anxious, and the aged. This uniquely human characteristic, the ability to communicate, is intimately related to nursing.

Burke's second characteristic of Man, the inventor of the negative, needs some explanation. In fact, it probably seems strange at first glance. Burke notes that all things are positive in nature.[7] There are no negatives. In other words, the negative is operationalized only when Man labels what is not: this is *not* a table, *not* a house, *not* the Waldorf. The negative is, according to Burke, "a function peculiar to symbol systems, quite as the square root of minus-one is an implication of a certain mathematical system."[8] Consequently, humans can perceive the negative; they can understand the terms "none," "nonexistence," "not happening." Humans are thus able to develop "Thou shall nots"—moral codes, negative rules for conduct, and laws that govern the relationships and functions of individuals as well as of institutions and professions. As children, we learn the "no-no"s early. The implications of the negative are quite germane to the heart of nursing. People can be aware of the possibility of their own nonexistence, or death, and they can plan for the implications that are inherent in this fact. We are concerned about this in nursing care of so many of our clients. So often death, nonexistence, or the negative, is a possible outcome of health problems. And human beings can develop future-oriented expectations of what can happen; we can be anxious about outcomes that may not happen. And we are concerned about this in nursing too. We all can remember a client whose leg did not have to be amputated, whose pregnancy did not happen, whose brain tumor was not malignant. To be aware of these possibilities is to suffer a uniquely human agony—and to experience the joy or grief of such things not happening is also uniquely human. This human characteristic, the awareness of negatives, is very relevant to nursing.

Burke next describes Man as being "separated from his natural condition by instruments of his own making."[9] By this, Burke means that Man, like all animals, is restricted to interacting within a limited area of his environment. Man can see only so far, hear sounds up to a limited distance, walk a certain distance in a given time. But because Man is capable of inventing tools, he is able to separate himself from the immediate environment and behave contrary to the natural laws and restrictions that are inherent in other life forms. Man is able to extend his own physical capabilities through the use of these tools, as in transportation by airplanes, communication by radio and television, food supply through the use of chemicals, and in making new compounds such as plastic. However, Man risks dangerous side effects in the quest for potential benefits. Man changes his relationship with the environment. This has relevance to nursing because so many of the health problems requiring nursing care are caused by Man's inventions. Our clients suffer the consequences in broken bones from automobile accidents, cancers from exposure to strange petroleum products, or other maladies from exposure to chemicals and radiation. Yet at the same time, taking a more positive view, so many of our clients live better (or at least longer) lives because of artificial heart valves and vessels made of plastic, artificial bones made of steel, and artificial kidneys made of tubes and filters. From this we can see that the human capacity to be separated from our natural condition by instruments of our own making is also truly relevant to nursing.

Burke next states that Man is "goaded by the spirit of hierarchy (or moved by the sense of order)."[10] This refers to all human incentives of organization and status. Man tends to organize life, relationships, and environment according to a particular perspective, criteria, or value system. Man tends to practice one-upmanship in relationships, and Man tends to seek power and status through control of others, through resources, through environment, or through all of these. This sense of hierarchy tends to result in conflict interpersonally, interprofessionally, and internationally. We encounter the spirit of hierarchy in each client-nurse relationship to some degree. In fact, it seems to penetrate the entire health-care system of which nursing is a part. This, then, is also believed to be a human characteristic of particular relevance to nursing.

Finally, Burke defines Man as being "rotten with perfection," meaning that human beings are aware of perfection, but cannot achieve it for long, if at all.[11] Burke sees this principle of perfection arising from Man's ability to symbolize. This is because language is intrinsically perfectionist. Man seeks "proper" names for things, and seeks complete satisfaction. Man strives for the "perfect" life. The rottenness of it in part is that we also speak of the perfect fool, the perfect villain. And this striving for perfection interacts with all the other innate characteristics that have been identified by Burke. He adds that there is a sort of

terministic compulsion to carry out the implications of one's terminology, quite as if an astronomer discovered by his observations and computations that a certain wandering body was likely to hit the earth and destroy us, he would nevertheless feel compelled to argue for the correctness of his computations, despite the ominousness of the outcome.[12]

And Burke also notes that there seems to be no built-in control that might prevent Man from carrying any set of activities or plans to the perfectly logical conclusion: the goal setting, the striving, the failing, the endless repetition of these actions that leads Man to the same fate. In nursing, we often see clients striving for some health goal that may be unrealistic in view of their present capabilities, resources, or environment. Consider, for example, the mother who wants the perfect baby but has a retarded child; the "A-type" personality salesman who wants the sales bonus but has a heart attack instead; the nursing service director who is going to have the perfect scheduling plan, but winds up with reality shock and burnout. We all think we know what it would be like if things worked perfectly. We are able to be future-oriented, to think and plan about how things would be if things functioned perfectly; and we tend to work and strive toward that end. But we also tend to experience frustration and disappointment because absolute control is rarely, if ever, possible. Perfection is illusionary and illusive.

The one characteristic that Duldt adds to Burke's list is that Man is self-reflective. In other words, Man is the only being capable of analyzing his own behavior, his own body functioning, and his own thinking and feeling processes. This has particular relevance to nursing because in the nursing process we strive to help clients understand their bodies and themselves so they may cope more effectively. This self-reflectiveness seems to be derived from Man's ability to symbolize, and it is also highly relevant to nursing.

Burke's lifelong interest has been the study of Man as a communicator. Thus he sees Man primarily as the user of symbols, and he notes that this has allowed Man to do certain things that are unique among all animals:

1. He can label things and talk about them when they are not present.
2. He can talk about the negative, that is, he can worry about what may not happen.
3. He can be aware of, know, and do things beyond his immediate environment.
4. He can develop categories and hierarchies according to some value or theme.
5. He can dream of how things could be if all were perfect.
6. He can talk about himself, reflect on his own behavior, and understand himself.

As cynical as Burke is with his descriptions of Man as "symbol-misusing" and "rotten with perfection," he is basically an optimist:

The best I can do is state my belief that things might be improved somewhat if enough people began thinking along the likes of this definition; my belief that, if such an approach could be perfected by many kinds of critics and educators and self-admonishers in general, things might be a little less ominous than otherwise.[13]

People in nursing need to think about Burke's definition of Man. And we need to have things seem a little less ominous or threatening for our future. Toffler states there has been more change in health care in the last five years than in the last fifty, and he indicates that the rate of this change can only be expected to increase in the next two decades.[14] In view of this, Burke's contribution to our definition of Man is central to the development of a knowledge base for the discipline and profession of nursing. It is not enough to borrow from other disciplines to define the focus of our discipline and service, the human being. We must define the human being or client as being able to think about himself—to worry himself sick. This is very human behavior.

Duldt developed the following set of phrases as an initial definition of Man, as derived from Burke's writings. The terminology she selected seems more appropriate to that commonly used in nursing, yet it retains much of Burke's intent.

Man is a living being capable of
symbolizing,
perceiving the negative,

transcending his environment by his inventions,
ordering his environment,
striving for perfection, and
self-reflecting.

These phrases are process-oriented and seem to incorporate more than
nursing scholars are now including under the bio-physical-psycho-
social definition of Man. Nevertheless, they still encompass all of this
traditional definition. For example, the term "living being" incorpo-
rates all the elements that are commonly classified as "biophysical"
aspects of Man. But in the new definition these characteristics are
seen as innate in Man regardless of his environment or his interactions with the environment. Specifically, this definition does not imply an adaptive process; there are no other intervening variables. The
nursing process can still be applied to all manner of intervening variables and interactions.

Characteristics

The definition of "human being" or client which Duldt ultimately
developed also shows the influence of Burke's work:

The client (human being) is an existential being who is the recipient
of nursing interventions and who has the following characteristics:

1. Living
2. Communicating
3. Negativing
4. Inventing
5. Ordering
6. Dreaming
7. Choosing
8. Self-reflecting

In other words, Man is an existential being who is a complex whole
composed of the interacting set of characteristics listed above. While
these characteristics are not necessarily unique to the species, these
are of particular concern to nursing. Thus, for nursing, these characteristics may be described as a set of elements that define the whole
human being.

Living.   Living refers to the ability of humans to function biologically
and physiologically as animalistic, viable entities. This biological

dimension is shared with other life forms and includes bodily, life-sustaining processes such as reproduction, assimilation, elimination, mobility, oxygenation, and so on. These processes are susceptible to injury, infection, malfunction, and ultimately death as human beings react to stressful stimuli, either external or internal. Like other life forms, a human being displays an orderly, sequential process of growth and development (and aging) that is influenced to some degree by that human being's lifestyle and environment (including such features as quality of nutrition, cleanliness of air, amount of exercise, and so on). As is true of all mammalian species, a human's existence depends upon interactions with members of his or her own species. Physiological responses to stimuli—such as flight or fight responses to danger or attack—are also shared in common with other life forms. In addition, the human being tends to share a sign system of nonverbal communication, also common to many other life forms, such as the sign systems that indicate territoriality, rejection, and acceptance.

Communicating. *Communicating* refers to the ability of humans to label things and to talk about them when they aren't present. As Burke puts it, humans are "symbol-using, mis-using" beings.[15] As a consequence, humans are able to build upon the learning, logic, and perceptions of predecessors and contemporaries through the written and spoken use of language. Using symbols enables Man to think abstractly, to use logic and argumentation, to solve problems, and to learn as well as communicate perceptions regarding phenomena observed concerning the physical environment, the self, and relationships with others. Humans are particularly capable of expressing feelings that arise from within as a response to perceptions. These expressions take many forms, from crying in grief or screaming in terror to expression in the arts of music and painting.

Negativing. *Negativing* refers to the ability of humans to talk about the symbolic negative: (− 1), no, none, not, not existing, not happening. Through this humans are able to develop moral codes, rules of conduct, and laws that govern the relationships and functions of individuals as well as of the environment. Humans can be aware of their own nonexistence, or death, and plan for the implications inherent in this fact. And because of this they develop certain expectations of what can happen in the future; they can be aware of the expected situation, which may not in fact happen.

Inventing. *Inventing* refers to the ability of the human being to devise tools that separate himself from the immediate environment.

Thus human beings can behave contrary to natural laws of the environment and the restrictions that are inherent in other life forms. The human being extends his own physical capabilities through the use of these tools in transportation (airplanes), communication (radio and television), chemistry (food preservatives), technology (plastics and computers), and so on. Unaided by these inventions, human beings can only hear a voice at a limited distance; with electronic communication equipment, one can hear a voice around the world, far out into space, and even into the future (by playing tape recordings at a later time). However, a human being risks dangerous side effects in the quest of potential benefits in changing his relationship with the environment. Some inventions have unanticipated effects, as in the case when insecticides used in food production cause covert poisoning in people and in animals. Thus the ability to invent has profound implications for human health.

Ordering.   Ordering refers to the ability of humans to develop categories and hierarchies according to some value or theme. In this way humans give structure and system to the environment and tend to organize life, relationships, and the environment according to a particular perspective or goal. Humans tend to practice one-upmanship in relationships and to seek power and status through control of others, of resources, of the environment, or of all of these. This sense of hierarchy tends to result in conflict.

Dreaming.   Dreaming refers to the ability of humans to consider things as they could be if all were perfect. Each human being has hopes, expectations, and dreams for the future. Each is able to think and plan about how things would be if all functioned perfectly and one tends to work and strive toward that end. And human beings are continually experiencing the frustration and disappointment as dreams become unattainable. Absolute control is rarely possible beyond brief periods for fallible humans, and perfection is illusionary and illusive.

Choosing.   Choosing refers to the ability of humans to consider numerous alternatives, compare implications for the future, and select the alternatives that tend to be the most desirable according to certain values and criteria. Thus human beings are able to make choices and control events in their lives, in their health, and in their circumstances. Human beings are also capable of being highly motivated to achieve short-term as well as long-term, even life-long, goals. And in the choosing, responsibility and accountability for the implications and results are also significant factors, ones that add a dreadful dimension to the whole process.

Self-reflecting. *Self-reflecting* refers to the ability of a human being to think and talk about his own self, his body, his behavior. This often involves such existentialist elements as "being," "becoming," "choice," "freedom," "responsibility," "solitude," "loneliness," "pain," "struggle," "tragedy," "meaning," "dread," "uncertainty," "despair," and "death." The act of self-reflection typically becomes salient during critical life situations.

Roles

A significant feature of Duldt's theory of humanistic nursing communication is that the definition of human being applies to both the client and the nurse. Both are human beings first. Both possess, given individual variances, all the characteristics or elements of being human. In this very real sense, they are equal, yet each is unique in individual expression of these characteristics. This definition, then, has implications not only for nurse-client relationships, but also for nurse-peer and nurse-colleague relationships. In addition, it has implications for the superior-subordinate relationships, such as that of the staff nurse and the head nurse or supervisor. Thus we now need to define more specifically the set of human beings or roles involved in Duldt's theory.

Nurse. The nurse is a human being who practices nursing, intervening through the application of the nursing process to develop a plan of nursing care for a specific client. The nurse possesses special educational and licensure credentials to qualify to practice nursing according to the dictates of the society in which he or she practices.

Client. The client is also a human being who is experiencing a critical life situation, potential or actual. This human being has a need for the special services of the nurse, and because of this he or she becomes the focus of the nursing process. The client is not necessarily to be construed as only one individual. Rather, the client can be seen as including the family of individuals providing the social support system for the client who is experiencing the critical life situation. Thus these individuals are also considered in the nursing process.

Peer. A peer of the nurse is defined as one who has equal standing in the same discipline and profession, that is, another nurse.

Colleague. A colleague is defined as a member of another discipline or profession, particularly those professionals with whom nurses coordinate, consult, and collaborate in the practice of nursing. Examples of colleagues of nurses include physicians, priests and similar religious advisors, and therapists.

Now that the "human being" has been defined, the next step is to consider, from a nursing perspective, what other concepts are uniquely relevant to it. For example, we would certainly need to describe how a human being happens to be in jeopardy—in other words, a *critical life situation.* Since a nursing theory by definition requires the inclusion of health, it would also seem reasonable to include this concept. And finally, a theorist needs to put the human being into some context, into an environment.

CRITICAL LIFE SITUATION

Man's life situation becomes critical when he perceives a threat to the state of his health, when his existential state of being is seen as being in jeopardy. For example, one's health is threatened to varying degrees by pregnancy, by the development of cancer, or in the event of accidents. Indeed, one's life may be in danger to some extent in each of these situations.

Significant changes in personal hygiene and health care are required to cope with critical life situations. The interaction of all the characteristics of human beings are believed to increase in intensity when one tries to adjust to such situations.

HEALTH

A human being's health is seen as his or her state of being, of becoming, and of his or her self-awareness. Thus health is perceived to be indicative of one's adaptation to the environment. While many view health as a continuum, extending from illness to wellness, Duldt views it as a free-flowing, existential state in a particular space, moving forward through time.

ENVIRONMENT

Duldt defines the environment as one's time/space/relationship context. Each human being exists in a particular time span in relation to the totality of the time continuum from past to future. Each person also exists in a particular spot in the universe; no one can be in two places at once. One has a particular relationship network with other human beings, a network that is unique to one's spot in time and space. Children and theorists often play the game of asking, "How would you like to have lived in another time?" One can think of the lifestyle of that period and decide. For example, how would you like to have lived in George Washington's time? It would mean wearing hand-carved, ivory false teeth, traveling by horse, having no refrigeration, and being bled when ill. Each individual has a very unique environment from which to view the world, and the uniqueness of this environment has special implications for the development of nursing-care plans for individuals.

Again, from a nursing perspective, the role and function of nursing as a profession and discipline need to be defined in order to account for the nurse's unique behavior as one human being interacting with other human beings who are experiencing critical life situations.

NURSING

We are now ready to define what nursing is about as a discipline as well as a profession. Where are we now in defining our discipline—our emerging discipline? According to the dictionary, a discipline is a field of study of human knowledge and inquiry. Generally, each discipline is identified by the distinct perspective it uses in viewing human beings and the environment in which they exist. Thus Donaldson and Crowley state:

In identifying disciplines and classifying them, we are dealing with the nature and structure of the whole of human knowledge. It should be kept in mind that the number and membership of the disciplines are not agreed upon and that there is no single, accepted organization of even the well-accepted disciplines. This is reflected in the diversity of organization of branches of learning in universities and colleges. The broadest classifications of disciplines depend upon a view of the inherent nature of all phenomena. A distinction on the part of the philosophers between the generality of natural phenomena and the particularity of human events leads to a distinction between such sciences as physics and sociology, which seek general laws for repeating behavior, and such disciplines as history, which focuses on unique events, or ethics, which deals with human choices and value orientations. . . . Among the sciences themselves, the biological sciences become distinct from physics and chemistry because they deal with the recognition of the phenomena of life and with living as opposed to non-living things.[16]

Donaldson and Crowley further state that there is a critical need to identify a structure for nursing as a discipline in our educational programs. In their review of nursing history, they identify three emerging themes that may serve to provide some structure. These are a concern for patterns and processes

1. of life, well-being, and optimum functioning of human beings— sick or well,
2. of human behavior in interaction with the environment in critical life situations; and
3. by which positive changes in health states are affected.[17]

Donaldson and Crowley propose that these themes suggest boundaries for the discipline of nursing, and Newman identifies criteria for nursing theories that are similar in theme.[18] Note the key term, *human beings*. This is the central focus of nursing.

Nursing as a discipline is currently perceived as being in the process of becoming a field of study and a profession. In other words, it is an emerging discipline. There seems to be a consensus among scholars that a theoretical body of knowledge is an essential element for this development. For example, Johnston notes the scarcity of theoretical and scientific giants in nursing's heritage upon which present-day nursing scholars might build.[19] Consequently, theories and models have been borrowed from other disciplines and professions to be applied with varying degrees of appropriateness to the nursing context.

Efforts toward achieving a theoretical basis in nursing have only occurred in the past fifteen years. We believe that nursing as an emerging discipline is at the preconceptual level of development in its theory building. Our concepts must be defined before our relationship statements can be developed. And relationships among concepts are the heart of a theory.[20]

As noted above, nursing has borrowed from other disciplines prior to these newer efforts. In fact, we have borrowed our definitions of the major concept of nursing, the human being. And among nursing scholars, there is still no generally accepted definition of nursing.

Orem, serving as chairman and editor of the Nursing Development Conference Group, presents a detailed analysis of the numerous definitions of nursing that occur in the literature.[21] Many of these definitions are specific to particular theories of nursing. In response to them, Duldt proposes the following definition to set boundaries as derived from Donaldson and Crowley's three themes found in nursing history:[22]

Nursing is the art and science of positive, humanistic intervention in changing health states of human beings interacting in the environment of potential or actual critical life situations.

Humanistic nursing denotes communication patterns and attitudes with which interventions are operationalized. It is communicating and relating interpersonally to clients in a manner that tends to operationalize the sort of communication in which the client senses warmth and acceptance and can report feeling good about his or her care. Consequently, humanistic nursing does not occur in just one particular place. Rather, it happens *between* human beings, between a nurse and a client.

There are implications for humanistic nursing in defining humans according to innate, existentialist characteristics. Because nurses are human beings, it would logically follow that nurses themselves would be subject to this definition. Since both clients and nurses share this common bond, then the relationship between clients and nurses would logically be on an equal basis, each respecting the other and showing a concern for the other's individual feelings, needs, worth, and responsibility.

We have the beginnings of a theory about how to humanize nursing by Patterson and Zderad that describes this "between" or "in-touchness" experience that happens between a nurse and a client.[23] They have derived this theory from the work of the humanistic philosopher, Martin Buber.[24] Thus Patterson and Zderad focus on the special phenomenon of interpersonal communication—on the warm, genuine, open relationship that is a positive validation of individual worth. They believe it to be essential to "releasing" people to develop to their fullest potential, to develop, as Patterson and Zderad phrase it, their "well-being" and "more-being." This may be that special part of nursing that is rewarding to nurses themselves. And to feel good about one's self, to feel acceptance, importance, and positive regard "releases" clients to heal faster.

The concept of "humanism" thus interacts with that of "nursing." Indeed, it may be the core of nursing. And the primary purpose of Duldt's theory is to give substance to communicating in a humanistic manner, to help nurses deliberately achieve the "I-Thou," the "in-between," or the "in-touchness" of relationships. In recognition of this, Duldt identifies a subset of elements of nursing. These elements are communicating, caring, and coaching.

Communicating

Communicating is the exchanging of a *message* between human beings. This message consists of *facts* and *feelings*, and it is conveyed in a manner involving attitudes and patterns of interactions, communicative behavior. It is through the ability to communicate that the nurse is enabled to use the nursing process—that is, by assessing, planning, implementing, and evaluating—as a systematic approach to the practice of nursing.

Caring

Caring involves valuing and touching. The nurse values the client and is concerned about that individual's well-being. Caring also involves touching in the sense of providing nursing care, the traditional sense of the "laying on of hands." Caring is feeling concerned and responsible for the client's health state.

Coaching

Coaching refers particularly to the teaching aspect of nursing. The nurse plans and implements the teaching and learning process within the total nursing process, and the nurse provides support and encouragement to the client as he or she strives to meet health goals. The nurse, as a private tutor, instructs, directs, and paces the client's progress toward health.

COMMUNICATION

We have defined communication, particularly interpersonal communication, as a dynamic process involving continued adaptation and adjustment between two or more human beings engaged in face-to-face interactions during which each person is continually aware of the other(s).[25] The content of their messages consists primarily of facts (information) and feelings (emotions).

Attitudes

Conceptually, the manner in which we communicate a message is called an "attitude." Thus attitude is defined here by Duldt as a mental position toward a person, fact, or state; it is our demeanor or predilection toward something. Furthermore, an attitude can be either humanizing or dehumanizing in nature. To communicate with a humanizing attitude generally means to be aware of the eight characteristics of a human being that have previously been presented. Conversely, to dehumanize is to ignore these characteristics. Thus these two types of attitudes can be thought of as occurring on a continuum as in Figure 18.

These gradations of the attitudinal dimensions of communication are believed to reflect the best available research and knowledge about

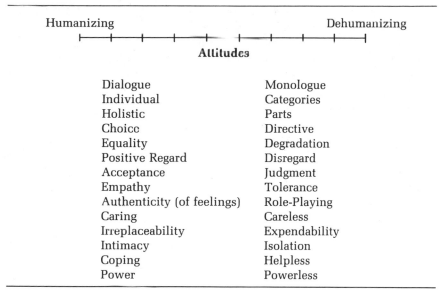

Figure 18. *The continuum of attitudes.*

how people interact and communicate in nursing. Such dimensions represent Duldt's attempt to identify humanizing attitudes of communication in which people are treated as people, not things. For more extensive definitions of these attitudes, the reader is referred to an earlier work.[26]

Interaction Patterns

A set of elements can be constructed for the specific interaction patterns of interpersonal communication behavior—that is, for how one communicates a message. This set includes communing, assertiveness, confrontation, conflict (resolution), and separation.

Communing

Communing refers to dialogical, intimate, humanizing communication that occurs between two or more people involved in nursing. It is a subjective event that happens "between" people and involves being aware of the other person's presence. It is "being there" and "being with." Dialogical communing is the element that makes nursing humanistic; conversely, if monological communication is used, nursing becomes dehumanizing. Typically, those involved in communing are the nurse and client, but it also includes the nurse and peers or the nurse and colleagues from other professions. Communing consists of three elements, which are the heart of humanistic communication: trust, self-disclosure, and feedback.

Trust is one person relying on another; risking potential loss in attempting to achieve a goal when the outcome is uncertain; and the potential for loss is greater than the potential for gain if the trust is violated.[27] Elements of trust include reliability, expertness, and dynamism (openness and frankness).

Self-disclosure is risking rejection in telling how one feels, thinks, and so on, regarding "here and now" events.

Feedback is describing another's behavior, beliefs, and so on, plus giving one's evaluation or feeling about the topic or issue.

Trust, self-disclosure, and feedback characterize communing, which is the core of a humanizing relationship. These three elements are seen as necessary to the development of a relationship in which each person is understood, cooperative, and satisfied. In other words, the relationship is valued by each person, and humanizing communication behavior occurs to a significant degree.

Assertiveness

Assertiveness is expressing one's needs, thoughts, feelings, or beliefs in a direct, honest, confident manner while being respectful of others' thoughts, feelings, or beliefs. If humanistic in nature, it is "asserting with authenticity."

Confrontation

Confrontation is providing feedback about another plus requesting a change in his or her behavior. If humanistic in nature, it is "confronting with caring."

Conflict

Conflict calls for a decision over an issue to which there is risk of loss as well as possible gain, in which there are two or more alternatives from which to choose, and in which one's values are involved. If humanistic in nature, it is "conflicting with dialogue."

Separation

Separation occurs at the end of a relationship. It may be due to change or choice, or to commitments outside the relationship. For example, a client may move to another area of the hospital or be discharged; similarly, a nurse may accept a promotion or move away. There is usually a change in proximity so that face-to-face interactions decrease or cease. If the separation is humanistic in nature, the individuals will be able to pick up the relationship easily—almost as if whatever time, distance, or circumstance caused the separation had not even occurred—should they meet again at a future time.

SUMMARY

All of the concepts of the humanistic nursing communication theory have now been defined. And in these definitions many sets of elements have been presented. An outline of the hierarchical arrangement of the concepts with the associated sets of elements is presented in Figure 19. These concepts constitute the terms used in Duldt's theory of humanistic nursing communication. In the next chapter, we shall consider how they are related to one another and the manner in which they interact.

Human Being
  Characteristics
    a. Living
    b. Communicating
    c. Negativing
    d. Inventing
    e. Ordering
    f. Dreaming
    g. Choosing
    h. Self-Reflecting

  Role
    a. Nurse
    b. Client
    c. Peer
    d. Colleague

Critical Life Situation

Health

Environment

Nursing
    a. Communicating
    b. Caring
    c. Coaching

Nursing Process
    a. Assessment
    b. Planning
    c. Implementation
    d. Evaluation

(cont.)

Figure 19. *Hierarchy of concepts and sets of elements in the theory of humanistic nursing communication.*

Communication
  Message
  a. Facts
  b. Feelings

  Attitudes

a. Humanizing	a. Dehumanizing
Dialogue	Monologue
Individual	Categories
Holistic	Parts
Choice	Directive
Equity	Degradation
Positive Regard	Disregard
Acceptance	Judgment
Empathy	Tolerance
Authenticity	Role-Playing
Caring	Careless
Irreplaceability	Expendability
Intimacy	Isolation
Coping	Helpless
Power	Powerless

  Interaction Patterns
  a. Communing (Trust, Self-Disclosure,
     and Feedback)
  b. Assertiveness
  c. Confrontation
  d. Conflict
  e. Separation

Figure 19—continued

NOTES

1. Abraham Maslow, *Toward a Psychology of Being* (New York: Van Nostrand, 1962).
2. Hans Selye, *The Stress of Life* (New York: McGraw-Hill, 1956).
3. Kenneth Burke, *Language as Symbolic Action: Essays on Life, Literature, and Method* (Berkeley: University of California Press, 1966), p. 3.
4. Ibid., pp. 1–16.
5. Ibid., pp. 3–4.
6. Ibid., p. 5.
7. Ibid., p. 9.
8. Ibid.
9. Ibid., p. 13.
10. Ibid., p. 15.
11. Ibid., p. 16.

12. Ibid., p. 19.
13. Ibid., p. 21.
14. Alvin Toffler, "Nursing Encounters of a Future Time," Keynote speech presented at the National League for Nursing Convention, Atlanta, Ga., April 30, 1979.
15. Burke, *Language as Symbolic Action*, pp. 3–9.
16. Sue K. Donaldson and Dorothy M. Crowley. "The Discipline of Nursing," *Nursing Outlook* 28 (February 1978):114.
17. Ibid., p. 114.
18. Margaret Newman, *Theory Development in Nursing* (Philadelphia: F. A. Davis, 1979), p. 2.
19. Dorothy E. Johnston, "Development of Theory: A Requisite for Nursing as a Primary Health Profession," *Nursing Research* 23 (September-October 1974):372–377.
20. See Chapter 8.
21. Dorothy E. Orem, ed., *Concept Formulation in Nursing*, 2nd ed. (Boston: Little, Brown, 1979).
22. Donaldson and Crowley, "The Discipline."
23. Josephine G. Patterson and Loretta T. Zderad, *Humanistic Nursing* (New York: John Wiley, 1976).
24. Martin Buber, *I and Thou*, trans. by Walter Kaufmann (New York: Scribner's, 1970).
25. Bonnie Weaver Duldt, Kim Giffin, and Bobby R. Patton, *Interpersonal Communication in Nursing* (Philadelphia: F. A. Davis, 1983), pp. 10–12.
26. Ibid., pp. 262–271.
27. Kim Giffin, "The Contribution of Studies of Source Credibility to a Theory of Interpersonal Trust in the Communication Process," *Psychological Bulletin* 68 (1967):104–120.

Relationship Statements *15*

Relationship statements describe how the concepts of a theory interact. To use an analogy, if the assumptions set the stage and the concepts are the actors, then the relationship statements are the script of a play. The actors follow the script, but sometimes that script doesn't do justice to their acting. In the same way, a theory may not organize, explain, and predict an event as we experience it in reality.

This, then, is the crucial test for Duldt's theory. How well does it match the reality of nurses' experience in communicating interpersonally with clients, peers, and professional colleagues? In the paragraphs that follow, we will present several relationship statements (hypotheses), some principles of communicating with a humanizing attitude, and a model of humanistic nursing communication.

Our major relationship statement is this: The degree to which one chooses to communicate with others with humanizing attitudes and interaction patterns, to that degree one will tend to operationalize humanistic nursing communication. More specific statements of the relationship are as follows:

1. The degree to which one receives humanizing communication from others, to that degree one will tend to feel recognized and accepted as a human being.
   a. While applying the nursing process, the degree to which a nurse is able to use humanizing communication, to that degree will the client, peer, or colleague tend to feel recognized and accepted as a human being.
   b. In a given environment, if a critical life situation develops for a client, to the degree the nurse uses humanizing communication attitudes and patterns while applying the nursing process, to a similar degree will the health of the client tend to move in a positive direction.
2. To the degree a nurse uses humanizing elements to communicate, he or she will tend to receive humanizing communication from peers, colleagues, and superiors.

221

Here the attitudes with which one communicates are used with the interaction patterns of communication. Thus a model can be presented (see Figure 20) that shows the specific patterns of communication within varying levels of closeness in a relationship. In this model, we see that trust, self-disclosure, and feedback represent the heart of humanistic communications, that is, of communing. These three elements also tend to be related: increase trust, and self-disclosure tends to increase, as does feedback; decrease any one of these three elements and the others also tend to decrease. Therefore the following relationship statements can be made:

3. To the degree that trust, self-disclosure, and feedback occur, to that degree humanizing communication or communing also occurs.
4. In the event one tends to experience dehumanizing communication—that is, monological rather than dialogical, categorical rather than individualistic, and so on—then one tends to move outward (on the model) to the next pattern of interaction. (See Figure 21.)

One tends to feel the pressure to express needs, thoughts, feelings, or beliefs with a little more definiteness and clarity when one hopes to move the relationship back toward the center toward trust, self-disclosure, and feedback; toward understanding, cooperation, and satisfaction. Thus the following relationships can be stated:

5. In an interpersonal relationship of trust, self-disclosure, and feedback, to the degree that dehumanizing communicative attitudes are expressed by another, to that degree one tends to use assertiveness as a pattern of interaction.
6. To the degree that assertiveness tends not to reestablish trust, self-disclosure, and feedback, and to the degree that dehumanizing communication attitudes continue to be expressed by another, to that degree one tends to use confrontation as a pattern of communication.

In the event use of assertiveness fails to move the interpersonal relationship toward the center, and thus the dehumanizing attitudes continue to be expressed, then one tends to move toward confrontation as an effective communication pattern. Therefore the following relationship statement can be made:

7. To the degree that confrontation tends not to reestablish trust, self-disclosure, and feedback, and to the degree that dehumaniz-

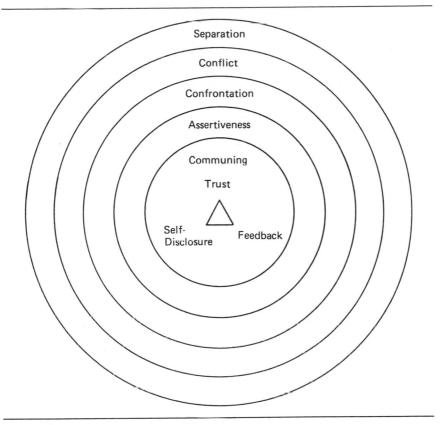

Figure 20. The communication patterns.

ing communication attitudes continue to be expressed by another, to that degree one tends to use conflict resolution as a pattern of communication.

Conflict situations may involve verbalization of polarization in regard to beliefs, values, and opinions. When this happens, cooperation may not be forthcoming, and meaningful dialogue may not occur. In fact, those involved in the relationship may become so dissatisfied that one or more of them choose to terminate it. Thus the following relationship statement can be made regarding the separation of individuals in a relationship:

8. To the degree that conflict tends not to reestablish trust, self-disclosure, and feedback, and to the degree that dehumanizing

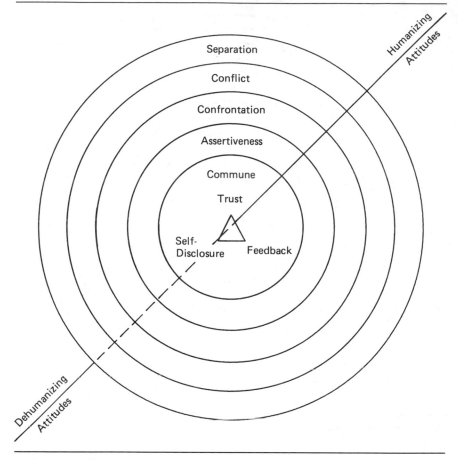

Figure 21. *The humanistic model of the interacting continuum of attitudes and patterns of communication.*

communication attitudes continue to be expressed by another, to that degree one tends to terminate the relationship by separation.

However, although separation occurs, it may not be the end of the relationship. Consider the following relationship statement:

9. To the degree that humanizing communication attitudes occur in a relationship, in the event of separation, the relationship can be resumed to the same degree of closeness regardless of the separation.

Individuals often speak of feeling so close to another person that, although they have been separated by distance and time, when they reunite it seems as if they had only been apart for a few minutes. Apparently individuals can feel so close to one another that they are able to pick up their conversations almost as if the separation had not occurred. Thus separation need not dictate the termination of a relationship. In fact, separation sometimes increases the value of a humanizing relationship.

Generally, as one moves away from the center of the model and away from the tripod of humanizing communication elements, dehumanizing patterns of communication tend to occur. However, it must be noted that in each of these circles the interaction pattern can also be either humanizing or dehumanizing. One can behave in a manner that generates the feeling of trust in others, but one can do so for the purpose of deceiving or manipulating. One can be assertive, but in an aggressive, disrespectful manner. One can confront in a punishing, hostile way. One can initiate conflict resolution in a vicious manner. One can separate from another in a way that terminates the relationship.

Because of all this, the humanistic communication model can be viewed in its totality as the dimensions of (a) interaction patterns and (b) attitudes, as seen in Figure 22. In other words, one has a choice. One may use all of the interaction patterns with varying degrees of humanizing or dehumanizing attitudes. And there is a wide range for each dimension. The assumption here, however, is that the nurse will choose to use the patterns of interaction in a humanizing mode, particularly when communicating with clients.

We must be aware, though, that the usual response is to communicate to another in the same manner in which that person communicates to us. Because of this principle of reciprocity, consider the following relationship statement:

10. The degree to which a nurse uses humanizing communication, to that degree will the nurse receive humanizing communication from others—clients, peers, colleagues, and superiors.

When one nurse approaches another in a respectful, considerate manner, the other nurse will tend to respond in a similar fashion. And the opposite is also true. When one speaks with anger, abruptness, and disrespect, the other person usually responds with anger, abruptness, and disrespect.

However, one has a choice. After all, each person is responsible for at least half of whatever is going on in a relationship. And the choices

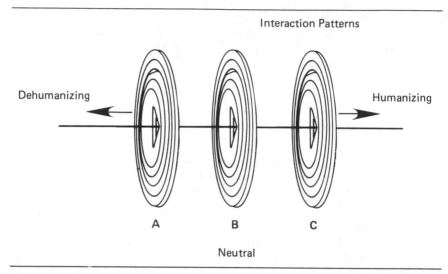

Interaction Patterns

Dehumanizing

Humanizing

A   B   C

Neutral

Figure 22. The humanistic model.

one makes are closely related to one's motives and expectations about the relationship. Thus, building on the knowledge of the dimensions of interaction patterns and attitudes, it can be seen that nurses have choice and thus have the potential for greater control of their relationships. Instead of randomly using interaction patterns and attitudes, nurses can communicate by design. From this, the following relationship statement can be made:

11. To the degree that one is *aware* of one's own *choices* (and motives) about interaction patterns and attitudes, to that degree one is able to develop communication skills and habits which tend to have predictable results in establishing, maintaining, and terminating interpersonal relationships.

It seems reasonable to propose that nurses who tend to deliberately choose humanizing attitudes in situations that in their judgment require assertiveness, confrontation, conflict resolution, or separation, will tend to establish, maintain, and/or end their interpersonal relationships in a humanistic way.

To return to Duldt's model, we should note that movement from the center to the outer circles may not necessarily be sequential. In fact, nonsequential movement may be more typical of reality. For example, a nurse may recognize a situation in which assertiveness is needed in

discussing an aspect of a client's care with a physician. Once assertiveness has been used, the interpersonal relationship is expected to
change. Conflict resolution involving bargaining and negotiating processes may become the next appropriate interaction pattern in order to
resolve differences of opinion and arrive at a decision regarding the
client's care. To learn only one pattern, such as assertiveness, although it may be helpful to some degree, tends not to be sufficient.
Thus nurses need to be able to recognize, categorize, and apply the
appropriate interaction pattern as well as attitude in the complex,
random, and multiple situations that arise in a typical day of nursing
practice.

It is also proposed that dehumanizing communications from others
can also be successfully handled by nurses through the use of the
interaction patterns and humanistic attitudes. Defensiveness, communication denial, verbal abuse, anger, and sexual harassment are all
communication patterns that present special problems for nurses.
Anger, for example, may occur at any level of the relationship model,
and it can be expressed in destructive (dehumanizing) or maintenance
(humanizing) modes.[1] The use of trust, self-disclosure, and feedback
is the basis of the maintenance mode of expressing anger. This mode
is the recommended way to receive another's angry expressions,
which are usually in the destructive mode; it is also a helpful mode
for expressing one's own anger. Communication denial, verbal abuse,
and sexual harassment also tend to require assertiveness, confrontation, conflict resolution, and separation.[2]

However, not all situations call for humanizing interaction patterns
and attitudes. A nurse may very wisely choose a dehumanizing attitude in talking to some individuals. For example, a young woman
nurse may choose to use dehumanizing attitudes and a confronting
interaction pattern to discourage a potential sexual harasser. After all,
if she chooses to terminate a relationship, then use of dehumanizing
attitudes and the conflict interaction pattern will probably hasten the
process toward separation. Nevertheless, in those contexts and relationships that are particularly relevant to providing care to clients, use
of humanizing attitudes with interaction patterns seems generally to
be preferable. Overall, it is important that the nurse be aware of the
range of choices that is available.

In summary, Duldt has proposed humanizing and dehumanizing
sets of attitudes that, when used with a set of interaction patterns, can
provide a considerable measure of control and predictability in interpersonal relationships. While human behavior is to a great extent
unpredictable because human beings have choice, it is nevertheless
through informed choice that unpredictability can be decreased for

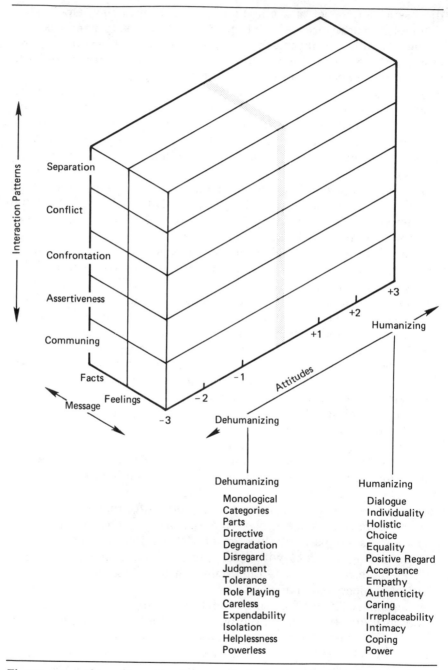

Figure 23. A three-dimensional research design for the humanistic nursing communication theory.

nurses who communicate in a manner each deems appropriate for the situation and the relationship.

A humanistic manner of communicating is preferable in most situations. It won't always work, and there are no guarantees. What Duldt is saying is that application of her theory of humanistic nursing communication will tend to result in outcomes that are predictable.

We must recognize that the operationalization of humanistic nursing communication is not seen as all sweetness, love, and laughter. The nurse who uses this theory most effectively is the one who displays a wide range of attitudes, both humanizing and dehumanizing; he or she is the one who displays skill in all of the interaction patterns. In doing so, the nurse need not be controlled by other people's communications through instinctive responding in like manner. Rather, the humanistic nurse is a thinking, planning, and choosing person who can deliberately select the attitude and interaction pattern most appropriate to the message content—that is, the facts and feelings to be communicated in specific situations, for need, for motives, and for relationships.

The research design suggested to test this theory is a three-dimensional one, as seen in Figure 23. And client-care situations can be selected to test the theory. For example, separation interaction patterns are necessary as clients achieve sufficient levels of health to move to new, more independent circumstances—that is, to step-down care areas or to their own homes. It is often necessary to provide certain instructions or information, that is, facts, to the client to assure his or her continued progress toward wellness. The attitude the nurse uses with the interaction pattern of separation in communicating these messages is expected to have an influence upon all the characteristics of the client as a human being.

The above represents the testing of only one pattern of interaction within the continuum of attitudes to view a holistic effect upon the human client (see Figure 24). Each pattern of interaction would need to be explored in a similar manner and replicated in many clinical nursing contexts to determine the validity of this theory. Methods of measurement and tools of data collection have already been developed for many of the concepts of this theory, although some adaptation would need to be made for nursing contexts. Certainly a long-term program of research is necessary to adequately test this theory.

Use of the concept "human being" as defined in humanistic nursing communication theory has potential for implementation in nursing curricula and in clinical nursing practice. The eight elements characterizing the unique features of humans are defined further to give our

Separation Pattern of Interaction

	Dehumanizing Attitude		Humanizing Attitude	
	Messages		Messages	
	Facts	Feelings	Facts	Feelings
Living				
Communicating				
Negativing				
Inventing				
Ordering				
Dreaming				
Choosing				

Characteristics of Human Beings as Areas of Assessment of Clients' Responses and Progress Toward Health

Figure 24. *A four-way interaction research design.*

readers an indication of how these elements can be developed. (See Figure 25.) For example, most nursing education programs have the nursing process as a major curriculum thread; most nursing service units within clinical health agencies have definitive statements regarding nursing care plans. Each of the eight elements of the human being could be considered in relation to the nursing process or nursing care plan. Furthermore, some curricula and nursing service units

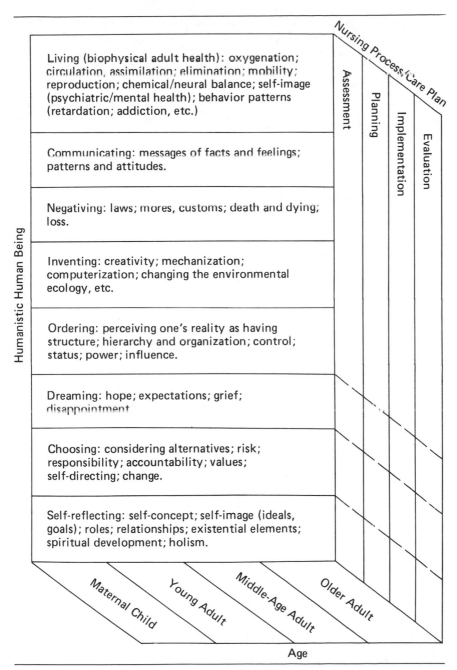

Figure 25. *Adaptation of definition of human being to nursing process and/or nursing care plan for nursing education and service.*

are organized about client age groups or some pragmatic set of categories, such as diagnostic groups, service, or clinical speciality. It is proposed that use of this definition of human being can be helpful in highlighting a larger scope—the wholeness of each client—thereby complementing and enhancing nursing practice.

In the next chapter we will consider the evaluation of Duldt's theory and speculate about its value to the discipline and profession of nursing.

NOTES

1. Bonnie W. Duldt, "Anger: An Occupational Hazard for Nurses," *Nursing Outlook* 29 (September 1981):510–518; Bonnie W. Duldt, "Anger: An Alienating Communication Hazard for Nurses," *Nursing Outlook* 29 (November 1981):640–644; Bonnie W. Duldt, "Helping Nurses to Cope with the Anger-Dismay Syndrome," *Nursing Outlook* 30 (March 1982):168–175; Bonnie W. Duldt, "Commentary: About Anger," *Nursing Outlook* 30 (March 1982):84–85.
2. Bonnie W. Duldt, "Sexual Harassment in Nursing," *Nursing Outlook* 30 (June 1982):168–174; "Letters to the Editor," *Nursing Outlook* 30 (November-December 1982):493–498; Bonnie W. Duldt, Kim Giffin, and Bobby R. Patton, *Interpersonal Communication in Nursing* (Philadelphia: F. A. Davis, 1983), pp. 217–244.

Evaluation 16

The next step in the process of developing a theory is to evaluate its practical value and applicability. As we have already seen, there are certain criteria that are helpful in making this determination. In this chapter, we will identify several of the most important ones in evaluating any theory, discussing each in terms of the theory of humanistic nursing communication. We believe this theory to be particularly applicable to the practice of nursing, and we will offer some support for this stand.

The first criterion to be met is that the theory needs to be clearly and simply stated. Often students of nursing have difficulty analyzing theories because the assumptions, definitions of concepts, relationship statements, and general discussions of each are all blended together, making it easy to become lost. In contrast, we believe we have presented Duldt's theory in an organized, logical sequence, giving each of its major aspects a separate chapter, so that students of nursing might readily understand it.

Duldt's statements of assumption describe the human being as an active (rather than reactive), process-oriented, symbolizing being who is capable of being influenced by communication events in the existential "here and now." These concepts are extensively defined so that operationalization and measurement are facilitated for future research purposes. The relationships between the concepts are stated in classic correlational, logical, deterministic or probabilistic forms so that research hypotheses, designs, and statistical tools can readily be developed and applied. Thus we believe that students and members of the nursing discipline will easily understand this theory and will tend to conduct research to test its validity.

A second criterion in evaluating a theory deals with the scope of the theory. In other words, what territory does it cover? Duldt's theory is intended to be applicable to nurse-client, nurse-peer, and nurse-colleague interpersonal communication occurring in all areas of nursing practice. It is a traditional "paradigm variation" that, according to

Reynolds, is a continuation of currently accepted theoretical perspectives, but with a change proposed in order to make the theory more useful and realistic.[1]

Duldt's theory is a paradigm variation of Martin Buber's "I-Thou" theory of communication.[2] The main distinction Buber makes is that human beings communicate differently with things ("I-It") than with people ("I-Thou"). Duldt's theory is also a paradigm variation of Patterson and Zderad's theory of humanistic nursing practice, which is itself a variation of the "I-Thou" theory.[3] We believe that Duldt's humanistic nursing communication theory differs from both of these in that:

1. It defines the human being in a manner most relevant to the realities of nursing practice.
2. It provides clearly stated assumptions, concepts, and relationship statements that are readily testable.
3. It provides a cohesive perspective of specific attitudes and interaction patterns that can be taught in schools of nursing.

Indeed, much of this theory is probably being taught currently in nursing curriculi in America, albeit in a fragmented manner.

A third criterion, or group of criteria, concerns the theory's applicability, generalizability, and agreement with known data and relevant research. We propose that Duldt's theory meets this group of criteria to a reasonable degree. First, in developing the theory, we have presented in another text discussions of theory and research that we believe represent the best information currently available about interpersonal communication.[4] In the present work, we have concentrated our efforts on ways in which normal, regular people tend to communicate and miscommunicate with one another. Moving from this broad base, we have focused on the interpersonal communication occurring in the professional role for nurses and have extensively developed selected areas of concern.

We propose that all interpersonal communication can potentially be helpful if it tends to be humanistic, as we have defined humanistic attitudes. To become therapeutic, a few additional patterns of communication are needed, such as those suggested by Carkhuff.[5] These also need to reflect humanistic attitudes in order to be effective.

The theory of humanistic nursing communication gives unique recognition to all of the negative, alienating, and dehumanizing encounters nurses experience with peers·and colleagues. It provides a structure for thinking of ways to cope with negative aspects of nursing practice, not just the "ought to," "should," and "must" some theorists tend to inappropriately impose on nurses' professional behavior. A review of most nursing theories shows that communication is included in them but is not developed extensively. It is thus anticipated that this theory of nursing communication can be used in association with other nursing theories to provide more specific guides to actions—that is, to the selection of patterns and attitudes to use in interpersonal relationships.

A fourth criterion in evaluating a theory is to estimate the theory's importance to the development of a discipline or an area of study. With some variations, numerous nursing scholars and leaders tend to support the idea of humanistic nursing. For example, Pilette describes the nurse as a "humanistic artist" in an existential philosophical context, and identifies the "nurse-client relationship as the cornerstone of the art of humanistic nursing."[6] She further states that:

Art, our most basic birthright, can be traced to the Biblical character Phoebe and her charitable manner of ministering to the Romans. This early intuitive art meant no more or less than comforting and caring for another human being. . . . In this humanistic era, it is fitting that nursing has reclaimed and updated its birthright. . . . The art of nursing has its deepest roots in the human care transaction and is confirmed in the dialogical process or "I-Thou" relationship.[7]

However, she further states that dialogue does *not* require special techniques.[8]

We take the opposite position and believe there is considerable evidence to support us. First, Carkhuff and Truax have found that didactic and experiential group training programs for professionals have resulted in increased levels of empathy, respect, and genuineness—all concepts that are included in Duldt's proposed theory.[9] Numerous special techniques or communication behavior patterns have also been described and classified as either promoting or destroying an interpersonal relationship—in other words, as either humanizing or dehumanizing.[10] We have focused particularly on those communication patterns that seem to be most relevant to the current practice of nursing—that is, communing, assertiveness, confrontation, conflict resolution, and separation.

Second, LaMonica specifically identifies positive attitudes as determinants of behavior congruent with humanistic nursing.[11] We have identified and emphasized sets of humanizing rather than dehumanizing attitudes as an essential factor in humanistic communication in nursing. This inherently humanistic quality of nursing has been described and discussed not only by LaMonica but also by Flynn,

Blattner, and Watson.[12] King and Gerwig also draw on humanistic education and the psychology of humanistic nursing education when they state that:

> Somewhere amidst all that equipment, behind all that SOAP charting, among all those nursing care plans, there is a human being—the patient. Have we become so involved in keeping up with the fast-paced technology and science of nursing and the hospital organizational routines, that we have lost sight of the art, the caring *humanistic* side of nursing? . . . It would appear that nursing is in need of a humanistic revolution, a return to the caring function of the nurse. It is our belief that a society weary of technology wants to put a stop to loss of identity and dehumanization, and that within our own profession, our patients desire a humane system of care that recognizes the humanity of us all as nursing priority number one.[13]

Many of the nursing authors identified above described the nurse and nursing as being inherently humanistic. And King and Gerwig even state that nursing educators have the responsibility of establishing models of humanistic education and learning so that this philosophy will ultimately permeate nursing practice.[14] Thus Lambertson has identified principles of professional education for nursing in colleges and universities that, according to King and Gerwig, have led to the current humanistic educational goals we know today.[15]

If nursing is indeed inherently humanistic, then interpersonal communication, which is the very process of humanizing, needs to be highly developed as a major concept in this discipline. And a humanistic definition of the human being, a definition that is unique to nursing and not borrowed from other disciplines, needs to be a consideration in each plan of nursing care. Giuffra stresses this, and Travelbee also moves to define the human being in terms somewhat similar to Duldt's.[16]

How is this to be done? One way is to develop communication as a focus by using Duldt's theory of humanistic nursing communication in association with other theories of nursing. Obviously, this theory cannot stand alone because it does not cover the entire territory of nursing. Rather, it serves to augment and enhance the realistic application of other theories that a nurse or faculty may choose to use. For example, many nursing theorists use communication as a concept, but do not significantly develop its definition. Instead, their focus tends to be elsewhere. For example, Roy focuses on adaptation, Orem on self-care, King on goal-oriented care, Newman on movement, and Yura and Walsh on the nursing process.[17] Yet in each of these theories, the interpersonal communication occurring between the nurse and the client is of paramount importance in order for the phenomenon of nursing to be operationalized.

General reviews of the nursing literature tend to show that the most basic skill in the assessment of the client's needs and the use of the nursing process, whether in the context of primary nursing or the most traditional delivery systems, is interpersonal communication. Yet research has shown that nurses tend to limit the communication of the client by ignoring cues and important disclosures. Thus Faulkner suggests that nurses not only need instruction in communication skills, particularly to become aware of the client's feelings, but also need assistance in dealing with the results of such communing so that neither the client nor the nurse is harmed by the experience.[18]

There are several ways in which the existential definition of the human being as proposed in Duldt's humanistic nursing communication theory can be used in nursing practice and education. In developing nursing care, the set of elements (living, communicating, negativing, and so on) can be used as an organizing principle for the entire care plan, or, more easily, it can be used as an additional check list to evaluate the comprehensiveness of care in meeting each need or solving each problem that is identified.

The problem-oriented charting and the SOAPs can continue and may be improved. After all, in nursing education, a theoretical framework based on needs, adaptation, or levels of care need not change, and the bio-physical-psycho-social organization of nursing content need not be set aside. Indeed, the humanistic description of the human being can be seen as a refinement of all of these perspectives of the client, one that is compatible with holistic nursing. It represents one further step toward the establishment of humanistic, primary nursing care as a dominant force in nursing as a discipline, as discussed and advocated by Fagin.[19]

NOTES

1. Paul Davidson Reynolds, *A Primer in Theory Construction* (Indianapolis: Bobbs-Merrill, 1971).
2. Martin Buber, *I and Thou*, trans. by Walter Kaufmann (New York: Scribner's, 1970).
3. Josephine G. Patterson and Loretta T. Zderad, *Humanistic Nursing* (New York: John Wiley, 1976).
4. Bonnie W. Duldt, Kim Giffin, and Bobby R. Patton, *Interpersonal Communication in Nursing* (Philadelphia: F. A. Davis, 1983).
5. Robert Carkhuff, *Helping and Human Relations: A Primer for Lay and Professional Helpers*, Vol. I, *Selection and Training* (New York: Holt, Rinehart and Winston, 1969); Robert R. Carkhuff, *Helping and Human*

Relations: A Primer for Lay and Professional Helpers. Vol. II, *Practice and Research* (New York: Holt, Rinehart and Winston, 1969).

6. Patricia Chehy Pilette, "The Nurse as a Humanistic Artist," in Arlyne B. Saperstein and Margaret A. Frazier, *Introduction to Nursing Practice* (Philadelphia: F. A. Davis, 1980), pp. 232–237.
7. Ibid., pp. 233–234.
8. Ibid., p. 237.
9. Robert R. Carkhuff and Charles Truax, "Training in Counseling and Psychotherapy: An Evaluation of an Integrated Didactic and Experiential Approach," *Journal of Consulting Psychology* 29 (1965):333–336.
10. Duldt, Giffin, and Patton, *Interpersonal Communication in Nursing.*
11. Elaine L. LaMonica, *The Nursing Process: A Humanistic Approach* (Menlo Park, Calif.: Addison-Wesley, 1979), p. 465.
12. Patricia Anne Randolph Flynn, *Holistic Health: The Art and Science of Care* (Bowie, Md.: Robert J. Brady, 1980); Patricia Anne Randolph Flynn, ed., *The Healing Continuum: Journeys in the Philosophy of Holistic Health* (Bowie, Md.: Robert J. Brady, 1980); Barbara Blattner, *Holistic Nursing* (Englewood Cliffs, N.J.: Prentice-Hall, 1981); Jean Watson, "The Philosophy and Science of Caring: Carative Factors in Nursing," in Patricia Anne Randolph Flynn, ed., *The Healing Continuum*, pp. 109–112.
13. Virginia G. King and Norma A. Gerwig, *Humanizing Nursing Education: A Confluent Approach Through Group Process* (Wakefield, Mass.: Nursing Resources, 1981), p. 19.
14. Ibid., pp. 32–33.
15. E. Lambertson, *Education for Nursing Leadership* (Philadelphia: Lippincott, 1958); King and Gerwig, *Humanizing Nursing Education*, pp. 25–28.
16. M. J. Giuffra, "Humanistic Nursing in a Technological Society," *Journal of the New York State Nurses' Association* 11 (March 1980):17–22; Joyce Travelbee, "Interpersonal Aspects of Nursing Concept: The Human Being," in Patricia Anne Randolph Flynn, ed., *The Healing Continuum*, pp. 71–72.
17. Sister Callista Roy, *Introduction to a Nursing Adaptation Model* (New York: Prentice-Hall, 1976); Dorothea E. Orem, *Nursing Concepts of Practice* (St. Louis: McGraw-Hill, 1971); Imogene M. King, *A Theory for Nursing: Systems, Concepts, Process* (New York: John Wiley, 1981); Margaret Newman, *Theory Development in Nursing* (Philadelphia: F. A. Davis, 1979); H. Yura and M. B. Walsh, *Nursing Process: Assessing, Planning, Implementing and Evaluation*, 2nd ed (New York: Appleton-Century-Crofts, 1973).
18. A. Faulkner, "Aye, There's the Rub—Communication Skills," *Nursing Times* 77 (February 19, 1981):332–336; J. Haywood, *Information: A Prescription Against Pain* (London: Royal College of Nursing, 1975); M. Johnson, "Communication of Patient's Feelings in Hospital," in A. E. Bennett, ed., *Communication Between Doctors and Patients* (New York: Oxford University Press, 1976), pp. 29–44.
19. C. M. Fagin, "Primary Care as an Academic Discipline," *Nursing Outlook* 26 (December 1978):750–753

Appendixes

Although one may develop categories to fit most of a phenomenon, some parts are often left over—like the dough remaining after the cookies have been cut out. And we have some "cookie dough" left over now that we have finished the book. In presenting such a complex subject as theory analysis, we need to point out some areas that we have treated lightly and that you, our readers, may wish to consider further.

One such area consists of the philosophical beliefs of nursing theorists and of nurses. One's philosophical stance influences to a considerable extent one's theoretical perspectives. Philosophy of scientific inquiry, empirical positivism, rationalism, and logical positivism are examples of some philosophies that may be of interest. There are also philosophies unique to academic disciplines, and eventually there may be a philosophy that is unique to nursing. Philosophical orientations provide significant and basic direction to the development of theories. You may find that knowledge of philosophical influences can be useful in categorizing and grouping nursing theories.

In this book we have urged our readers to use a form of theory analysis sheet that divides each theory into four major categories. Thus Appendix A is included here to summarize the points we have recommended for consideration in each column. However, it is important for our readers to recognize that other factors and more detailed outlines may also be used as the basis of theory analysis. In fact, a critic is free to select the categories for analysis and the criteria for evaluation. For example, the rhetorical critic Kenneth Burke set up six categories for the analysis of any symbolic situation: agent, act, agencies, scene, purpose, and attitude.[1] In turn Fisher's application of this analysis provided fascinating insights to a multiple murder and suicide.[2]

In a similar fashion, we can study organizations with the following set of categories: who says what to whom, when, and with what effect. Journalists and historians use categories very much like these. And in nursing, categories that involve even more details are now being suggested. For example, Kim offers "conceptual domains" as a means of organizing and relating concepts.[3] And Stevens uses ways of perceiving and processing information.[4]

We suggest that you give such approaches careful consideration. In the process, perhaps you will find that one or more of them can be incorporated into the one that is presented here. Ultimately, however, we recommend that you select one single analysis format and use it consistently so that you can compare one theory with another and make judgments about their usefulness. This represents a high level of sophistication in the analysis of theories, and it is our hope that you will be able to achieve it.

Following the sample format in Appendix A, you will find other theory analysis sheets that have been prepared by Duldt and some of her nursing theory students. Thus two analyses of the theories of Watson and King are included in order to demonstrate the differing perspectives of the nurses who were critiquing the theories. Each analysis sheet shows how the theory was understood by each individual nurse-analyst. We must remember, though, that the burden of clearly communicating what is intended ultimately rests with the theorist. In comparing the analysis sheets, you will find that some are more complex than others; this difference may be a reflection of either the theory or the analyst's perceptive discrimination.

Finally, we risk redundancy by stressing the following. It is imperative that nurse researchers know and understand the theory being tested. And the research needs to contribute to the body of knowledge about nursing practice. Our study of nursing theories and our research must influence nursing care practices and make a difference in how well we can predict the outcomes of nursing actions and interventions.

NOTES

1. Kenneth Burke, *A Grammar of Motives* (Berkeley: University of California Press, 1945).
2. Jeanne Y. Fisher, "A Burkean Analysis of the Rhetorical Dimensions of a Multiple Murder and Suicide," *Quarterly Journal of Speech* 60, no. 2, (April 1974):175–189.
3. Hesook Suzie Kim, *The Nature of Theoretical Thinking in Nursing* (Norwalk, Conn.: Appleton-Century-Crofts, 1983).
4. Barbara J. Stevens, *Nursing Theory: Analysis, Application, Evaluation* (Boston: Little, Brown, 1979).

List of Appendixes

Appendix A. Sample Theory Analysis Sheet

Theorist:

Theory:

Phenomenon Observed:

Analysis by:

Reference:

Assumptions	Concepts	Relationship Statements	Evaluation
Definition: accepted as true without testing.	*Definition:* a term or word used to classify and describe a phenomenon; a timeless, impersonal, and abstract idea; serves as a norm.	*Definition:* logical or natural association between two or more concepts within a set of assumptions.	*Definition:* to fix a value, significance or worth of something by careful analysis and study.
Function: Set parameters for theory; a frame that does not change or move.	*Function:* labels phenomena within a frame of assumptions.	*Function:* provide meaning to concepts, promote understanding, and predict outcomes. Show movement of concepts.	*Function:* to rate the degree of significance and give direction for revision.
Topics:	Topics:	Topics:	Criteria:

1. Goal and nature of science.	1. Ways to define:
	  a) Dictionary
	  b) Synonyms
	  c) Derivation
	  d) Operational definition:
	    1) experimental
	    2) measurable
	    3) administrative
	    4) evaluation
	  e) Scope and limitations
	  f) accomplishment, role, function
	  g) analogies and metaphors
	  h) authority quotes
	  i) sets of elements
		1. Relates all concepts in theory.	1. Shaw and Costanzo (sociology)
			  a. Necessary:
			    1) logical consistency
			    2) agrees with known data
			    3) testable
			  b. Desirable
			    1) clear and simple
			    2) economical
			    3) consistent with related theories
			    4) matches experiences
			    5) useful

2. Nature of human being.		2. Statements follow forms conducive to stimulate research—i.e., logical, analytical, correlational, deterministic, probabilistic.	

3. Nature of human motivation.			2. Newman (nursing)
			  a. focuses on life processes
			  b. patterns of processes related to health
			  c. concerns health promotion

4. Nature of truth, reality; epistomology.			
5. Source of influence on humans; reality, society, genetics, environment, past.		3. Use of model that includes all concepts and promotes understanding of relationships among concepts.	

6. For nursing: man, health, environment (society), and nursing.		4. Theorist draws on eristic thinking to build arguments to support relationship statements.	3. Stevens (nursing)
			  a. nursing acts
			  b. patient
			  c. health
			  d. interrelationship of the above

7. Source of assumptions.	2. Uses concepts of nursing paradigm—i.e., Man, health, environment, and nurse.		
8. Level of analysis: cells or societies.			

4. Duldt and Giffin (communication and nursing)
   a. Assumptions
      1) human being
      2) state or trait theory
      3) static or process reality
      4) any unstated assumptions
   b. Concepts
      1) definition complete (9 ways)
      2) operationalization
      3) measurable
      4) borrowed
   c. Relationship statements
      1) pattern used to state provides direction for research
      2) describe, explain, predict, and control
      3) easily converted to hypothesis
      4) intuitively realistic
   d. General
      1) parsimony
      2) applicability and generalizability
      3) explains and covers phenomena
      4) agrees with known data
      5) internally consistent
      6) research stimulated; supportive of or refutes theory
      7) importance to discipline and/or profession
      8) use in other disciplines
      9) criticism of others

Appendix B. Roy's Nursing Theory of Adaptation

Theorist: Sister Callista Roy	**Analysis by:** Bonnie W. Duldt
Theory: Nursing Theory of Adaptation	**Reference:** Sister Callista Roy and Sharon L. Roberts, Theory Construction
Phenomenon Observed: Nursing Practice	in Nursing: An Adaptation Model (Englewood Cliffs, N.J.: Prentice-Hall, 1981).

Assumptions	Concepts	Relationship Statements	Evaluation
Derived from the Systems Model:	1. *Nursing:* A science, a discipline, and a health care practice that focuses on the assessment, diagnosis, and treatment (interventions) of clients having health problems within the domain of nursing.	1. If the client is an adaptive system, and if the goal of adaptation is reached when the focal stimuli are within the client's adaptation level, then nursing intervention involves manipulating focal, contextual, and residual stimuli so the person can cope with the stimuli.	1. *Parsimony:* Roy's theory is distributed over numerous references. It contains a reasonable number of concepts, but numerous relationship statements. There is also some overlapping of concept definitions. For example, "the coping mechanism" refers to either one or both, or to parts of both of the adaptive modes and internal processor system.
1. A system is a whole which functions as a totality due to interdependence of its parts (subsystems) for some purpose.	2. *Health:* A continuum from illness to wellness. It is determined by the client's adaptive level and stimuli falling within or without the zone of that adaptive level. If stimuli fall inside the zone, then adaptive responses occur; if outside, then maladaptive responses occur.	2. If unusual stress or weakened coping mechanisms make a client's usual attempts to cope ineffective, then the person needs a nurse.	2. *Scope:* Roy's theory covers a broad territory—all of nursing practice. It excludes information about the nurse, except implicitly, and focuses entirely on the client. There is, however, some slippage of conceptualization of the human being: the bio-physio-psycho-social set is the organizing principle for examples rather than the adaptive modes and internal processor systems of human living systems being the organizing principle or genre of theoretical examples.
2. Living systems are comprised of matter and energy organized by information into subsystems arranged in a hierarchy.	3. *Environment:* The source of internal or external stimuli; either focal, contextual, or residual. A series of suprasystems, systems, and subsystems; it is always in the process of change.	3. The coping mechanism (regulator and cognator) acts in relation to the adaptive modes.	Follows the eristic thinking in its arrangement of logic, but in concepts, sets of elements, etc., however, definitions are not adequately developed in relation to the processes used in eristic thinking.
3. Information is the content (matter and energy) exchanged with the environment of a living system.	4. *Human being:* An open, adaptive system receiving input from the environment, both internal and external. Can be seen as an individual, a family, a community or a society and includes both nurse and client.	4. If energy is freed from inadequate coping attempts, then it can be utilized to promote healing and wellness.	3. *Limitations:* Roy's theory borrows concepts from the theories of other dis-
4. Processing of information is communication, a necessary factor in adaptation.	5. *Adaptive responses:* These function to achieve the human living system's goals of survival, growth, reproduction, self-mastery, and wellness. Responses can be either effective or ineffective.	5. If the coping mechanism (regulator and cognator) is ineffective, then ineffective behaviors result:	
5. Living systems are composed of subsystems arranged in hierarchy.		a. If the regulator system is ineffective, then physiological data (blood pressure, pulse, respiration etc.) will reflect the degree of ineffectiveness.	
6. Living systems seek to maintain balance or equilibrium through an adaptive (or feedback) system of variable standards and negative feedback.			
7. Adaptive, living systems maintain equilibrium to ever higher levels of organization.			

8. A system is a process, having no beginning or ending. (Implicit)

9. Creativity is possible when the system fails and adjustments become necessary for survival of the system. (Implicit)

Derived from Stress-Adaptation Theories:

10. The goals of adaptation of the total system are survival, growth, reproduction, and mastery as well as high-level wellness.

11. A human being is an adaptive being who, rather than being a victim of the environment, has control over resources and is capable of making choices.

12. In changing environments, human beings encounter adaptation problems, especially in situations of health and illness.

13. Living systems are subject to stress due to internal or external stimuli or stressors.

14. Living systems have an adaptation level which is the sum of three classes of stimuli: focal, contextual, and residual.

15. The adaptation level of a living system establishes the parameters for positive responses to stimuli.

16. Each living system must

6. *Central processing subsystem:* This processes all stimuli, stressors, or input. It consists of:

(a) Regulator system, which consists of physiological functions (neural, endocrine, chemical, and "target tissue"), linked to regulator and cognator systems by "connectives" of the internal processing system.

(b) Cognator system, which enables one to grasp reality and manipulate change through the use of such symbol systems as information processing, learning, judgment, and emotion.

7. *Adaptive modes:* These are either effectors or activators of adaptive responses, linked to regulator and cognator systems by "connectives" of the internal processing system. The four subsets of adaptive modes are labeled physiological, self-concept, role function, and interdependence.

8. *Nursing process:* This is a systematic method of practice to promote the client's adaptive modes and effective adaptation and to manipulate stimuli falling within the client's zone of adaptation. It consists of:

(a) Assessment: the collection of data on modes and stimuli, the development of a nursing diagnosis and the placement of the client on a health status continuum.

(b) Intervention: the mutually agreed upon goals identified and the resultant action taken by the nurse, based on choices and options offered to the client.

b. If cognator system is ineffective, then the degree of ineffectiveness will be reflected in the degree of the client's awareness of needs, ability to identify goals, ability to select means to goals, and the degree to which goals are attainable. (Implicit)

6. If the behavior of the client has been clearly specified, then the nurse can write goals of expected outcomes mutually agreed upon by both nurse and client.

7. Behaviors will tend to be adaptive if the client can keep securing adequate information about the environment, maintain satisfactory internal conditions for action and for processing information, and maintain autonomy.

8. The adaptation level varies with the pooled effect of focal, contextual, and residual stimuli or stressors.

9. If the effort to overcome stress is not sufficient, the coping mechanisms will be activated to produce greater responses.

10. The nurse makes judgments about the effectiveness of adaptive response behaviors based on a value hierarchy of goals to be achieved and on the long-term effectiveness of these behaviors.

11. For the regulator system:

a. The degree of internal and

ciplines without redefining. (Example: target tissue and reinforcement.) It follows the holistic view of the human, but excludes the spiritual, humanistic, and existential aspects of being human. Man is defined as a survival-oriented, behaviorist (condition-response), amoral, living system. Its concepts have yet to be operationalized and its measurement methods determined.

4. *Applicability:* Roy's theory provides an excellent, broad theoretical perspective with which other theories illuminating small scopes of theoretical territory can be used. For example, a developmental theory is used in pediatric care setting and a communication theory to enrich nurse-client dialogue section. It is compatible with most medical models of pathophysiology and related theories, and taxonomies. It is also useful in fostering communication between nurses and physicians. The theory arose out of Roy's own clinical practice experiences.

5. *Generalizability and agreement with known data:* Roy presents numerous theories and research from other disciplines as well as nursing to provide a foundation for the theory. It has great potential generalizability.

6. *Relevant research:* There is no relevant research, and Wagner encountered difficulty in using the theory in clinical practice. Use in ICU areas is believed to require considerable revision of the approach.

(continued on next page)

Assumptions	Concepts	Relationship Statements	Evaluation

balance its use of adaptive energy. (Implicit)
 	
17. Some stress is necessary for a living system's optimal adaptation. (Implicit)
 	
18. Nurses can identify a client's degree of optimal adaptation and maladaptation due to excessive or prolonged stress. (Implicit)
 	
19. Nurses can classify on a continuum of health (wellness to illness) the client's level of adaptation and maladaptation. (Implicit)
 	
20. A living system's reaction to stress is limited to the smallest amount of adaptation necessary to maintain a steady state, thus conserving adaptive resources or energy. (Implicit)
 	
Derived from Nursing:
21. Human beings are holistic, adaptive, living systems, capable of making choices and being responsible for their own bodies. (Implicit)
 	
22. Human beings have the ability to represent reality and manipulate it for themselves and for others by spoken or unspoken words.
 	
23. The goal of nursing is to
		external stimuli influences the degree of physiological response.
		  b. The degree to which nerve pathways are intact influences neural output effectors.
		  c. Chemical and neural inputs influence the responsiveness of the endocrine glands to harmonally influence target organs in a manner to maintain equilibrium.
		  d. responses of the body alter the stimuli.
		  e. The magnitude of stimuli may be so great that the adaptive systems cannot maintain the body's equilibrium.
		
		12. For the cognator system:
		  a. The optimum amount of clarity of input stimuli influences the adequacy of the cognator system's functioning.
		  b. Intact pathways and perceptual/information-processing apparatus influence the adequacy of cognator systems.
		  c. The degree of accuracy of the cognator processes influences the effectiveness of psychomotor response choices.
		  d. The psychomotor response choices will be activated through intact effectors.
			7. *Importance to the Discipline:* Roy's theory is a significant contribution. It focuses on what nursing is and not what it should be. It can provide a basis of organizing nursing knowledge for curricula. Furthermore, it emphasizes the nursing diagnosis, the development of nursing as a role, and the extensive data base that exists for nursing decisions and interventions.

promote adaptation of human beings.

24. The intended outcome of nurses' promoting clients' adaptation is high-level wellness.

25. The client is an active participant in nursing care.

26. Nursing interventions are directed toward manipulation of the environment.

e. Effector activity produces responses at the adaptive level determined by the cognator system.

f. The level of adaptive responses to stimuli alters the stimuli.

13. The meaning of perception will influence the body response.

14. The regulator and cognator systems are associated through the process of perception.

15. If stimuli cause behavior, then stimuli must be changed to change behavior.

16. The client is enabled to reestablish equilibrium to the degree the nurse can accurately assess, diagnose, and implement changes in the stimuli. (Implicit)

Appendix C. Duldt's Theory of Humanistic Nursing Communication

Theorist: Bonnie W. Duldt

Theory: Humanistic Nursing Communication

Phenomenon Observed: Interpersonal Communication between Nurse and Client, Peers and Colleagues

Analysis by: Bonnie W. Duldt

References: Bonnie Weaver Duldt, Kim Giffin, and Bobby R. Patton, *Interpersonal Communication in Nursing: A Humanistic Approach.* (Philadelphia: F.A. Davis, 1983); the present text.

Assumptions	Concepts	Relationship Statements	Evaluation
Derived from Philosophy: 1. Human beings exist in a "here and now" existential context from which there is no escape. 2. Human beings are continually concerned with such existential elements as: being, becoming, choice, freedom, responsibility, solitude, loneliness, pain, struggle, tragedy, meaning, dread, uncertainty, despair, and death. 3. All elements of existential being and the communication imperative are salient issues to be dealt with in critical life situations. 4. Growth and change arise from within the individual and to a considerable degree depend upon one's choice. 5. The nurse shares with the client all characteristics of being human. *Derived from Communication:*	*Human being:* Man is a living being capable of symbolizing, perceiving the negative, transcending his environment by his inventions, ordering his environment, striving for perfection, making choices, and self-reflecting. *Characteristics:* 1. *Living:* Able to function biologically and physiologically as an animalistic, viable entity. 2. *Communicating:* Able to label things and to talk about them when they aren't present. 3. *Negativing:* Able to talk about the symbolic negative (-1, no, none, not), make rules (laws regarding the "thou shalt not's"), worry about what may not happen, and consider his own nonexistence. 4. *Inventing:* Able to be aware of, know, and do things beyond his or her immediate environment, to invent things, and to change his relationship to the environment. 5. *Ordering:* Able to develop categories and hierarchies according to some	1. The degree to which one receives humanizing communication from others, to that degree one will tend to feel recognized and accepted as a human being. a. While applying the nursing process, the degree to which a nurse is able to use humanizing communication, to that degree will the client, peer, or colleague tend to feel recognized and accepted as a human being. b. In a given environment, if a critical life situation develops for a client, to the degree the nurse uses humanizing communication attitudes and patterns while applying the nursing process, the health of the client tend to move in a positive direction. 2. To the degree a nurse uses humanizing elements to communicate, he or she will tend to receive humanizing communications from peers, colleagues, and superiors.	1. *Clearly stated:* This theory is presented in an organized, logical sequence, and is readily understood. Assumptions are stated according to widely recognized academic patterns. Its concepts are extensively defined. The relationship statements are presented in a pattern that covertly implies research designs and statistical analysis. This theory is expected to stimulate more research efforts than the theories of Buber and of Patterson and Zderad. 2. *Scope:* This theory is applicable to nurse-client interpersonal communication in all areas of nursing. It is also applicable to nurse-peer and nurse-colleague relationships. As a paradigm variation of Buber's "I-Thou," and of Patterson and Zderad's humanistic nursing theory, this theory provides a more readily testable and measurable approach to abstract concepts. It also incorporates the writings and research of Burke (1966), Jourard (1971), Egan (1970, 1971), Berlo (1960), Patterson and Zderad (1976), Yura and Walsh

6. Survival is based on one's ability to communicate with others in order to share feelings and facts about the environment and ways of coping.

7. The environment is a "booming, buzzing" world of strange sensations that must be sorted out to determine which are most important; this sorting is achieved through communication with other people.

8. The need to communicate is an innate imperative for human beings.

9. Due to innate fallacies, human beings use and misuse all capabilities, especially the ability to communicate. An example is speaking to a human being as a thing rather than a person.

10. The way in which a person communicates determines what that person becomes.

11. Interpersonal communication is a humanizing factor that is an innate element of the nursing process (assessment, planning, implementation, and evaluation) and of the communication that occurs between nurses and clients, nurses and peers, and nurses and professional colleagues.

12. Evaluation of a person's own communication skills is subjec-

value of theme; gives structure and system to one's environment.

6. *Dreaming:* Able to dream of how things could be if all were perfect; expectations, hopes for future.

7. *Choosing:* Able to consider numerous alternatives, implications for the future.

8. *Self-Reflecting:* Able to think about and talk about self, reflect on own behavior and understand self, body, behaviors, etc. Conscious of the existential elements (see assumption #2).

Roles:

Nurse: A human being who practices nursing, intervening through the application of the nursing process to develop a plan of nursing care for a specific client or group of clients. The nurse possesses special educational and licensure credentials as required by society.

Client: A human being who is experiencing a critical life situation, potential or actual. He or she has need of the services of the nurse and is the focus of the nursing process. The client can also be seen to include the support system of family, friends, and so on.

Peer: A nurse having equal standing or status to another nurse.

Colleague: A member of another profession with whom nurses coordinate and collaborate in the practice of nursing—that is, physicians, administrators, ministers, and members of

3. To the degree that trust, self-disclosure, and feedback occur, to that degree humanizing communication or communing also occurs.

4. In the event one tends to experience dehumanizing communication—that is, monological rather than dialogical communication, categorical rather than individualistic, and so on—then one tends to move outward (on the model) to the next pattern of interaction. (See figure.)

5. In an interpersonal relationship of trust, self-disclosure, and feedback, to the degree that dehumanizing communication attitudes are expressed by another, to that degree one tends to use assertiveness as a pattern of interaction.

6. To the degree that assertiveness tends not to reestablish trust, self-disclosure and feedback, and to the degree that dehumanizing communication attitudes continue to be expressed by another, to that degree one tends to use confrontation as a pattern of communication.

7. To the degree that confrontation tends not to reestablish trust, self-disclosure or feedback, and to the degree that dehumanizing communication attitudes continue to be expressed by another,

(1973), Kierkegaard (1957), Maslow (1954), Mead (1934), Rogers and Truax (1971), Sartre (1957), Patton and Giffin (1977), Giffin and Patton (1974), and others.

3. *Applicability:* This theory is realistic in that it recognizes the ways in which nursing and health care systems are dehumanizing to nurses, clients and others. However, it emphasizes the choice of the nurse in using communication patterns that tend to be humanizing. It is an "is" theory, not a "should" theory. This is also a "state" theory in that it assumes that communication "here and now" can change the future.

4. *Generalizability and agreement with known data:* The theory is derived from a broad base of communication theory and research. It brings together information often taught in nursing curricula and puts it into a cohesive perspective that is intended to be more readily understood and used by nurses.

The theory is unique in that it recognizes the negative, unpleasant encounters nurses often have in clinical practices, and it provides a framework for developing modes of coping with dehumanizing communications.

5. *Research support for the theory.*

a. On trust by K. Giffin (1967). Extensive support from speaker credibility

(continued on next page)

Appendix C—Continued

Assumptions	Concepts	Relationship Statements	Evaluation
tive; each individual must make his or her own decisions and choices about communication behavior and choose to change, depending upon his or her ability to utilize feedback. Derived from Nursing: 13. The purpose of nursing is to intervene to support, maintain, and augment the client's state of health. 14. A human being functions as a unique, whole system responding openly to the environment. Specific to the Theory: 15. Health, satisfaction and success in a person's life and work—in other words, that person's state of being—is derived from feeling human. 16. Due to the bureaucratic and complex nature of the present health-care delivery systems, there is a tendency for clients and professionals to be treated in a dehumanizing manner and to relate to one another in a dehumanizing manner. 17. Humanizing patterns of communication can be learned and can enhance the nurse's awareness of and sensitivity to the client's state of being and of becoming.	health care professions and community service agencies. Nursing: The art and science of positive, humanistic intervention in the changing health states of human beings interacting in the environment of critical life situations. Its elements are communicating, caring, and coaching. Nursing process: This involves assessment, planning, implementation and evaluation. Health: One's state of being; of becoming; of self-awareness. It is indicative of one's adaptation to the environment. Environment: One's time/space/relationship context. Critical life situation: A situation in which there is a perceived threat to one's health state, in which one's existential state of being is salient, as in cancer, childbirth, accidents, and so on. Communication: A dynamic interpersonal process involving continual adaptation and adjustments between two or more human beings engaged in face-to-face interactions during which each person is continually aware of the other(s). A process characterized by being existential in nature, involving an exchange of meaning, concerning facts and feelings, and involving	to that degree one tends to use conflict resolution as a pattern of communication. 8. To the degree that conflict tends not to reestablish trust, self-disclosure, and feedback, and to the degree that dehumanizing communication attitudes continue to be expressed by another, to that degree one tends to terminate the relationship by separation. 9. To the degree that humanizing communication attitudes occur in a relationship, in the event of separation, the relationship can be resumed to the same degree of closeness regardless of the separation. 10. The degree to which a nurse uses humanizing communication, to that degree will the nurse receive humanizing communication from others—clients, peers, colleagues, and superiors. 11. To the degree that one is aware of one's own choices (and motives) about interaction patterns and attitudes, to that degree one is able to develop communication skills and habits which tend to have predictable results in establishing, maintaining and terminating interpersonal relationships.	research in the field of speech communication. b. Jourard (1971), Egan (1970, 1971) on self-disclosure and feedback. c. Grant (Duldt)(1977) found that anger expressed in the maintenance mode tends to increase group cohesiveness and maintain relationships between nursing task members; the destructive mode of expressing anger tends to destroy relationships, decreasing productivity and group attraction. d. Duldt (1982) identified the "anger-dismay" syndrome as a complex of behaviors nurses tend to display when receiving destructive-mode anger from others, especially from superiors. e. Duldt (1982) found that training workshops in communicating alienating messages, especially anger, decreases feelings of guilt and increases awareness of alienating patterns of communication. Role-playing and rehearsal also assist nurses in improving coping. 6. Importance to the Discipline: Nursing is being described as humanistic by many nurse authors, but few nurse theorists have reflected this in their theories of nursing. This theory is not intended to stand alone, but explains in detail only the phenomenon of communication. It is intended to serve with other nursing theories to augment and enhance the realistic appli-

18. The goal of the humanistic nurse is to break the communication cycle of dehumanizing attitudes and interaction patterns. replacing these with attitudes and patterns that humanize.

19. Interpersonal communication is the means by which the nurse becomes increasingly sensitive to and aware of the client's state of being, of the dynamic relationship between the client and his or her environment, and of the client's potential.

dialogical communing. It contains the following set of attitudes:

Humanizing		Dehumanizing
	continuum	
Dialogue		Monologue
Individual		Categories
Holistic		Parts
Choice		Directives
Equality		Degradation
Positive Regard		Disregard
Acceptance		Judgment
Empathy		Tolerance
Authenticity (of feelings)		Role-Playing
Caring		Careless
Irreplaceability		Expendability
Intimacy		Isolation
Coping		Helpless
Power		Powerless

Humanistic communication involves an awareness of the unique characteristics of being human.

Dehumanizing communication ignores the unique characteristics of being human.

Set of Interaction Patterns of Communication:

Communing: Dialogical, intimate communication between two or more people; the heart of humanistic communication.

1. Trust: One person relying on another on another, risking potential loss in attempting to achieve a goal, when the outcome is uncertain; and the potential for loss is greater than for gain if the trust is violated.

cability of other theories in clinical nursing. For example, the patterns of interactions and the attitudes of this theory would enhance nursing theories involving the nursing process and the communicating occurring with its operationalization. Also, the patterns of interaction and attitudes of the nurse are a significant aspect of therapeutic touch theory and would augment this theory as well.

(continued on next page)

Appendix C—Continued

Assumptions	Concepts	Relationship Statements	Evaluation
	2. *Self-disclosure*: Risking rejection in telling how one feels, thinks, and so on, regarding "here and now" events.		
	3. *Feedback*: Describing another's behavior, beliefs, and so on, plus giving one's evaluation or feelings.		
	4. *Assertiveness*: Expressing one's needs, thoughts, feelings or beliefs in a direct, honest, confident manner while being respectful of others' thoughts, feelings or beliefs: "asserting with authenticity."		
	5. *Confrontation*: Providing feedback about another plus requesting a change in his or her behavior: "confronting with caring."		
	6. *Conflict*: Requires a decision over an issue in which there is risk of loss as well as possible gain, in which two or more alternatives can be selected, and in which one's values are involved: "conflicting with dialogue."		
	7. *Separation*: The end of a relationship due to change, choice, or outside commitments: "separation with sadness."		
	Note: Trust, self-disclosure, and feedback represent the center of humanistic communicating—the central tripod.		

WORKS CITED IN APPENDIX C

Berlo, David K. 1960. *The Process of Communication.* San Francisco: Rinehart.

Burke, Kenneth. 1966. *Language as Symbolic Action: Essays on Life, Literature, and Method.* Berkeley: University of California Press.

Duldt, Bonnie W. 1982. "Helping Nurses to Cope with the Anger-Dismay Syndrome." *Nursing Outlook* 30 (March):168–175.

Egan, Gerard. 1970. *Encounter: Group Processes for Interpersonal Growth.* Belmont, Calif.: Brooks/Cole.

Egan, Gerard, ed. 1971. *Encounter Groups: Basic Readings.* Belmont, Calif.: Brooks/Cole.

Giffin, Kim. 1967. "The Contribution of Studies of Source Credibility to a Theory of Interpersonal Trust in the Communication Process." *Psychological Bulletin* 68:104–120.

Giffin, Kim, and Bobby R. Patton. 1974. *Personal Communication in Human Relations.* Columbus, Ohio: Charles E. Merrill.

Grant (Duldt), Bonnie Weaver. 1977. "Anger, Cohesiveness, and Productivity in Small Task Groups." Ph.D. dissertation. University of Kansas, Lawrence.

Jourard, Sidney M. 1971. *The Transparent Self.* 2nd ed. New York: Van Nostrand.

Kierkegaard, Soren Aabge. 1957. *The Concept of Dread,* translated with introduction and notes by Walter Lowrie, 2nd ed. Princeton: Princeton University Press.

Maslow, Abraham H. 1954. *Motivation and Personality.* New York: Harper and Brothers.

Mead, George H. 1934. *Mind, Self, and Society.* Edited by Charles W. Morris. Chicago: University of Chicago Press.

Patterson, Josephine G., and Loretta T. Zderad. 1976. *Humanistic Nursing.* New York: Wiley.

Patton, Bobby G., and Kim Giffin. 1977. *Interpersonal Communication in Action.* New York: Harper and Row.

Rogers, Carl R., and Charles B. Truax. 1971. "The Therapeutic Conditions Antecedent to Change: A Theoretical View." In *Encounter Groups: Basic Readings,* edited by Gerard Egan. Belmont, Calif.: Brooks/Cole.

Sartre, Jean-Paul. 1957. *Existentialism and Humanism.* Translated and with an introduction by Philip Mairet. Brooklyn: Hastings House.

Yura, H., and M. B. Walsh. 1973. *The Nursing Process: Assessing, Planning, Implementing, and Evaluating.* 2nd ed. Norwalk, Conn.: Appleton-Century-Crofts.

Appendix D. Newman's Nursing Theory of Health

Theorist: Margaret A. Newman

Theory: Nursing Theory of Health

Phenomenon Observed: The Nature of Health

Analysis by: Chris Burd, R.N., B.S.N., graduate student, University of North Dakota

Reference: Margaret Newman, *Theory Development in Nursing* (Philadelphia: F. A. Davis, 1979).

Assumptions	Concepts	Relationship Statements	Evaluation
Explicit (p. 56):	*Explicit (p. 59):*	*Explicit (p. 60):*	1. *Parsimony:* Exceptionally short and concise. Not very clear; could use more description of the concepts.
1. Health encompasses conditions heretofore described as illness or pathology.	1. Movement: awareness of self, property of matter, brings about change.	1. Time and space have a complementary relationship.	
2. These "pathological" conditions can be considered a manifestation of the total pattern of the individual.	2. Time: measures consciousness.	2. Movement is a means whereby space and time become reality.	2. *Scope:* Very broad—so broad, in fact, to be nonspecific to nursing.
	3. Space: is not described (can it be?).		3. *Applicability:* Newman suggests this theory be used as a prerequisite to nursing practice as opposed to a grand nursing theory. That is, if nursing had a grasp on the interrelationships of these four concepts, then the search for the one, unifying grand nursing theory would not be necessary.
3. The pattern of the individual that eventually manifests itself as pathology is primary and exists prior to structural or functional changes.	4. Consciousness: expansion is what life (and consequently health) is all about (p. 66).	3. Movement is a reflection of consciousness.	
	Implicit:	4. Time is a function of movement.	
4. Removal of the pathology in itself will not change the pattern of the individual.	5. Man.	5. Time is a measure of consciousness.	
5. If becoming "ill" is the only way an individual's pattern can manifest itself, then that is health for that person—that is, getting well, integration of self.	6. Health.	*Implicit:*	This writer feels that the theory provides a wonderful, broad background to be aware of when developing further theory, but cannot be used alone to unify nursing practice, it is much too general and could be applied to any number of situations. Actually, Newman seems to want to achieve this feeling of universality and common ground in all mankind.
	7. Holism: patterns, not separate functions.	6. If nursing is to be practiced, then there must be an understanding of the phenomena of health as a part of the dynamic interaction of time, space, movement, and consciousness.	
6. Health is the expansion of consciousness.	8. System.		
Implicit:			4. *Relevant Research:* Mention is made of Susman and Evered's work on "Action research." Newman feels a new research strategy is needed for developing theories of practice within
7. The process of the theory is never complete (p. 4).			

8. The development of the theory needs the conceptualization of health (p. 4).

9. Nursing science is the process of facilitating the health of Man (p. 7).

10. Life is composed of the energy of matter and motion [p. 23].

11. "Perfect" health is nonexistent (p. 55).

12. Man is a living system (p. 69).

13. Approximations of reality help science to be successful without the necessity of having to understand everything at once.

14. Man is a holistic being.

15. The focus of nursing science is the phenomenon of man (p. 2).

living, open systems. Piaget is referred to in connection with his statements on the concepts of time and movement. No research is proposed for testing the theory, which is a very broad one. Its concepts would defy operationalization because they could mean different ideas to each person who reads them.

5. *Internal Consistency:* States that *Man* should be the focus of nursing science, then goes on to use concepts of time, space, movement, and consciousness, leaving the reader to make the "jump" to reality, fitting in Man where he belongs.

6. *Abstractness:* Very abstract, an exercise in mental gymnastics, so to speak. The reader is required to attempt to fit the pieces of the nursing paradigm—*Man, health,* environment, and *nurse*—into their place in the cosmos. Not a bit concrete.

However, Newman's lead-in with several chapters on nursing theory development in general was quite good, as were her final pages on what is needed in research to be able to test systems that address holism.

Appendix E. Watson's Theory of Caring as a Basis for Nursing

Theorist: Jean Watson

Theory: Caring as a Basis for Nursing

Phenomenon Observed: Use of Carative Factors in All Nurse-Client Relationships

Analysis by: Chris Burd, R.N., B.S.N., graduate student, University of North Dakota

Reference: Jean Watson, *Nursing: The Philosophy and Science of Caring* (Boston: Little, Brown, 1979).

Assumptions	Concepts	Relationship Statements	Evaluation
1. Nursing is a therapeutic interpersonal process (preface).	*Carative Factors Concepts:* 1. Humanistic-altruistic system of values (maturity) (p. 12).	1. If scientific values are not congruent with humanistic values, then discrepancy between theory and practice occurs (p. 8).	1. *Parsimony:* a. Concepts, assumptions, and relationship statements are clear throughout; some are well developed. b. *Most of the concepts and assumptions are clearly outlined and explicitly identified.*
2. Nursing is a humanistic and scientific discipline as well as an academic and clinical one (preface).	2. Instillation of faith and hope (healing power of belief) (p. 14).	2. If a nurse forms person-to-person ("I-Thou") relationships, then the health and higher-level functioning of the patient is promoted (pp. 18–19).	2. *Scope:* Global—all nurse-client interaction is covered; this is the basis for all of nursing as a discipline.
3. Caring is only demonstrated and practiced interpersonally (pp. 8–9).	3. Cultivation of sensitivity to self and others (empathy) (p. 17).	3. If a nurse has high levels of congruence, empathy, and nonpossessive warmth, then a helping-trust relationship will occur. These facilitative dimensions further another's self-exploration and self-experiencing leading to constructive action (p. 38).	3. *Applicability:* a. Seems to set down what nurses have known intuitively all along. b. Provides a formal framework for the caring involved in nursing. c. Can be used universally in any nursing practice.
4. Caring promotes health and growth of individual and family (pp. 8–9).	4. Helping-trust relationship (congruence, empathy, nonpossessive warmth, effective communication) (pp. 26–40).	4. If there is no help-trust in a relationship, then a potentially harmful relationship may occur for both nurse and patient (p. 39).	4. *Generalizability:* a. (Chinn & Jacobs) "potential generality." b. Weak on research as of yet.
5. Caring consists of causative factors that result in the satisfaction of certain human needs (pp. 8–9).	5. Promotion and acceptance of the expression of positive and negative feelings (Rosenberg's affect/cognition) (p. 46).	5. If feelings influence behavior, nursing may be attentive to feelings and to responses to ill-	5. *Concepts Defined:* a. Each concept developed, but to varying degrees. b. None is fully described according to the nine ways of defining a concept.
6. Caring responses accept a person not only as he or she is now, but as what he or she may become (pp. 8–9).	6. Use of scientific problem-solving for decision-making (body of knowledge to serve as foundation for practice: requires theory and scientific method) (p. 60).		
7. Caring is more "healthogenic" than curing. Caring is complementary to curing (pp. 8–9). Treatment of disease constitutes only 10% of all health care issues (p. 220).	7. Interpersonal teaching: learning ("without learning, there has been no teaching") (p. 79).		
	8. Provision for a supportive, protective, and/or corrective mental, physical, sociocultural, and spiritual environment (external variables, safety,		

8. The practice of caring is central to nursing.

9. A caring environment is one that offers the development of one's potential while allowing the person to choose the best action for himself or herself at a given point in time (pp. 8–9).

10. Caring has existed in every society (p. 6).

11. Nursing's most important goal is the promotion of self-actualization (p. 201).

12. The human being is motivated by needs on multiple levels (cited throughout book).

13. The human being is in a continuous process of development (cited throughout book).

14. The human being is holistic (cited throughout book).

15. The human being experiences development both as an individual and/or as part of a group or family (p. 245).

16. Stress is related to many physical and social disorders (p. 224).

17. Development is inherently tied to health and holistic care (p. 246).

---

ness in order to promote health (p. 48).

6. If carative factors are combined with science (problem-solving method), then holistic nursing care will occur (p. 58).

7. If carative factor of scientific method is used, then nursing can expect, even predict, positive health outcomes (p. 66).

8. Helping-trust is related to interpersonal teaching-learning. Rogers: learning depends on the personal relationship between teacher and learner (p. 75).

9. If amount of accurate information is increased, then patient will experience decreased stress and increased health (p. 72).

*10. Use of all the carative factors (science of caring) will result in the promotion of holistic health. Use of carative factors results in disease prevention as opposed to curing (p. 78).

11. If humanism plus faith-hope plus sensitivity, then support of the human being (p. 83).

12. If helping-trust plus acceptance of positive and negative feelings, then potential for support, protection, and correction

---

privacy, comfort, clean and aesthetic surroundings) (pp. 81–100).

9. Assistance with the gratification of human needs (lower order/higher order/biophysical, psychosocial/psychophysical/intra-inter personal) (pp. 105–206).

10. Allowance for existential-phenomenological factors (unique experiences of the individual, value of the total personal context) (pp. 205–214).

Other Concepts:

11. Stress: change (part III).

12. Developmental conflict (part III).

13. Loss (part III).

14. Care versus cure (pp. 8–9).

---

c. Many concepts are grounded in other behavioral theories.

6. *Patterns of Relationship Statements:*
a. Relationship statements are not labeled as such.
b. "If . . . then" wording can be inferred between various concepts.
c. No hint is given as to which statistical tools could be used in researching the statements.
d. Statements do propose to explain and predict, however.

7. *Importance to Discipline:*
a. Goals are congruent with goals of nursing.
b. Definitely pertains to nursing practice—pervasive, global, affecting all nurse-client interaction.

8. *Limitations/Exclusions:*
a. All concepts come up short on operationalization. For example: "Additional study, practice, and research are required for nursing to include the gratification of higher order needs as a carative factor—but for now it suffices to establish the conceptual basis for human needs as a pertinent concern of nursing as the science of caring and the resultant movement toward health" (pp. 201–203).
b. No empirical data cited; very weak on research throughout.
c. Some of the carative factors were well developed and described and well related to other theories, but others were weakly developed—especially the first three carative factors of humanis-

(continued on next page)

Assumptions	Concepts	Relationship Statements	Evaluation
		of the human being (in primary prevention sense) (p. 83). 13. If scientific method plus interpersonal teaching-learning, then support, protection, and correction of human being (p. 83). 14. Use of several carative factors concurrently is sometimes indicated in practice of another carative factor (pp. 182, 191, 192). For example, the carative factor interpersonal teaching-learning can assist with the cognitive part of self-actualization (p. 199). *15. No one factor can be effective alone (p. 214). †16. If no existential-phenomenological perspective, then incomplete understanding of health and human being coping with illness (p. 214). *17. If study, practice, and research into health-illness behavior of persons coping with stress (change, developmental conflict, and loss plus the caring intervention of nurses that promotes humanism, health, and quality living), then illness prevention, health promotion, positive outcomes, and a higher level of wellness (p. 217).	tic-altruistic system of values, instillation of faith and hope, and cultivation of sensitivity to self and others. This is particularly important because Watson sees these as the foundation or "essence" of caring from which the others develop. d. Science of caring will never be an exact science, "such as physics" (p. 58). e. Not clear in part III why author focused on stress and change, developmental conflict, and loss as acting upon the human being. One wonders what went into the choice of these three concepts over all other influences on the human organism. f. Probably not knowingly, Watson has implied that nurses are superhuman. No address is made to nurses' limitations as human beings. Are all nurses able to deal with *all* the needs, conflicts, stresses, and losses of patients just by virtue of the label "nurse"? Several of the carative factors seem almost impossible to operationalize or to teach to prospective nurses. For example, development of humanistic-altruistic system of values. Such a value system would hinge upon an entire lifetime's pattern on the part of the nurse, influenced by personal factors such as ethics, religious beliefs, and culture—factors that may overlap into nursing practice but which can-

not be specifically developed at will for a nursing career. Such a concept can be presented and grasped intellectually but cannot be expected to be internalized automatically

18. If increase in stress, developmental change, loss, then increase in illness (p. 218).

19. If holistic care, then decreased stress and increased health-maintenance by human being.

*20. If nurse intervening aware of stress, developmental change, loss, then increase of relevance of health care to daily living (not addressed only to illness symptoms) (p. 218).

21. If stress causes illness, then increased difficulty in diagnosis and treatment (p. 224).

*Relationship statements central to entire theory.
†Comment: Needs this revision to conform to criteria for relationship statements (B. Duldt).

Appendix F. *Watson's Theory on the Philosophy and Science of Caring*

Theorist: Jean Watson

Theory: The Philosophy and Science of Caring

Phenomenon Observed: Nursing Intervention with Caring to Move Clients Toward Optimal Health

Analysis by: Karan Rondeau, R.N., B.S.N., graduate student, University of North Dakota

Reference: Jean Watson, *Nursing: The Philosophy and Science of Caring* (Boston: Little, Brown, 1979).

Assumptions	Concepts	Relationship Statements	Evaluation
1. Caring can be effectively demonstrated and practiced only interpersonally.	1. *Nursing:* Being established as a discipline that has great knowledge and understanding of human behavior. The foundation is caring.	1. The quality of one's relationship with another person is the most significant element in determining help effectiveness.	1. *Parsimony:* Although many points and concepts are brought up as the theory is developed, the general thread is this: If caring is used as a nursing intervention, then optimal health will result. Many of the individual concepts did not relate; however, they are all tied to caring.
2. Caring consists of carative factors that result in the satisfaction of certain human needs.	2. *Environment:* A person is never without an environment or a biological system that affects his or her behavior. The set of variables of the environment are: a. Comfort b. Stress c. Privacy d. Safety e. Cleanliness and aesthetics	2. The degree to which one's needs are gratified, to that degree one is able to grow and develop to potential.	2. *Scope:* The author identifies a broad scope to cover all areas of nursing practice and to reach every level of nursing practitioner. She does a very good job of including all areas of nursing, differentiating between nursing as caring and medicine as curing.
3. Effective caring promotes health and individual or family growth.		3. If one's higher-order needs are met, one is less often preoccupied with the lower-order needs.	3. *Applicability:* This theory is unlimited. The prerequisite to most of nursing is caring.
4. Caring responses accept a person not only as he or she is now, but as what he or she may become.	3. *Human/Humanities:* People and their emotional response to experiences, as well as individual and family differences and uniqueness.	4. If primary nursing intervention occurs around those three human conditions (stress-change, developmental conflicts, and loss), then nursing health care will be relevant to the daily circumstances of living, not simply to illness symptoms and problems.	4. *Generalizability:* See comments under scope. This is such a far-reaching concept, I cannot imagine a situation to which it could not be applied.
5. A caring environment is one that offers the development of potential while allowing the person to choose the best action for him or herself at a given point in time.	4. *Health:* People in good health can meet the daily expectations of their family, job, and social role. Health is a process of adapting, coping, and growing that goes on from conception to death.		5. *Agreement with known data:* I feel the author utilized different disciplines to bring in studies, graphs, and models to identify and clarify her points and stand. Since there is not
6. Caring is more healthogenic than is curing. The practice of caring integrates biophysical knowledge with knowledge of human behavior to generate or promote health and provide ministrations to those who are	5. *Caring:* This includes the following: a. Humanistic-altruistic value system	5. If objective diagnosis and treatment are ineffective in promoting and maintaining health, then health professionals, health industries and society must realize the need for a different em-	

ill. A science of caring is therefore complementary to the science of curing.

7. The practice of caring is central to nursing.

8. Caring has existed in every society. A caring attitude is not transmitted from generation to generation, but is transmitted by the culture of the profession as a unique way of coping with its environment.

9. There is a discrepancy between theory and practice or between the scientific and artistic aspects of caring.

10. Biophysical needs are considered to be a given and known focus of nursing care.

11. Need is a requirement of a person, which if supplied results in diminished distress. The gratification of a human need is necessary for growth and development.

b. Instillation of faith-hope

c. Sensitivity to one's self and others

d. Development of a helping-trust relationship

e. Promotion and acceptance of the expression of positive and negative feelings

f. Systematic use of scientific problem-solving method for decision-making

g. Promotion of intrapersonal teaching-learning

h. Promotion of supportive, protective, and/or corrected mental, physical, sociocultural, and spiritual environment

i. Assistance with gratification of human needs

j. Allowance for existential-phenomenological forces; accounting for courage and miraculous happenings in the existence of others

6. Congruence: An openness with feelings and attitudes; genuineness.

7. Empathy: The nurse's ability to experience the other person's private world and to communicate some significant degree of understanding.

8. Nonpossessive warmth: Unconditional regard.

9. Communication: Cognitive, affective, and behavioral responses used to convey a message to another person.

10. Human needs: A holistic dynamic

phasis (new knowledge and new skill in educating people, promoting or facilitating behavior and lifestyle change and helping people) to become their own best health care providers.

6. If health wellness is the concept that guides the practice of nursing and the science of caring, then new, nonmedical models must be continually explored. (Note: New emphasis on self-care and self-control are necessary for high-quality health, coping, and adaptation to stress, so that individuals are the best providers of health care for families.)

much nursing theory to build on, this could not be used. However, the author presents a point with which to follow nursing process for suggestions of evaluation and research.

6. *Relevant research:* The studies of Roy and King were acknowledged in the text. The author frequently pointed out the lack of nursing research and the need for such projects.

7. *Importance:* Even though the author did not do a good job of making clear the relationships between concepts, (she just related caring to each one) this theory is basic to nursing. She did the profession a service by writing it down for reference. The information will provide a solid foundation from which research can be launched. It is a very useful theory and book. The theory is concrete and is easy, enlightening reading. My only criticism is that it is sometimes hard to keep the overall point in mind as you become wrapped up in the details.

My model interpretation is simply:
Nurse + Client + Caring + Environment = Health

(continued on next page)

Appendix F—Continued

Assumptions	Concepts	Relationship Statements	Evaluation
	approach including the following set of elements: a. Biophysical b. Psychophysical c. Psychosocial d. Intrapersonal Low-order needs are: a. Food and fluids b. Elimination c. Ventilation d. Activity-inactivity e. Sexuality High-order needs are: a. Achievement need: behavior aimed at satisfaction of an internal standard of excellence b. Affiliation need: people need people for help and companionship. c. Self-actualization need: a movement toward health and self satisfaction; the highest quality of life. 11. *Stress:* Factors that are dependent on a person's lifestyle, behavior, personality, and social environment. 12. *Development Conflicts:* Affect one's ability to cope with the stress of health and illness. 13. *Loss:* Can only be understood in terms of what it means to the person involved. A loss to one may not be a loss to another.		

Appendix G. King's Goal Attainment Theory of Nursing

Theorist: Imogene M. King

Theory: Goal Attainment Theory of Nursing

Phenomenon Observed: Nursing Practice Goals

Analysis by: Kathleen Sonnesyn, R.N., B.S.N., M.S., graduate student, University of North Dakota

Reference: Imogene King, A Theory for Nursing: Systems, Concepts, Process. (New York: John Wiley, 1981).

Assumptions	Concepts	Relationship Statements	Evaluation
1. Individuals are social beings. 2. Individuals are sentient beings. 3. Individuals are rational beings. 4. Individuals are reacting beings. 5. Individuals are perceiving beings. 6. Individuals are controlling beings. 7. Individuals are purposeful beings. 8. Individuals are action-oriented beings. 9. Individuals are time-oriented beings. 10. Perceptions of nurse and of client influence the interaction process. 11. Goals, needs, and values of nurse and client influence the interaction process.	1. *Man:* Man is a social, sentient, rational, reacting, perceiving, controlling, purposeful, action-oriented, and time-oriented being (p. 143). Man is an open system exhibiting permeable boundaries permitting an exchange of matter, energy, and information (p. 69). 2. *Nursing:* Nursing is a process of human interactions between nurse and client whereby each perceives the other and the situation. Through communication they set goals, explore means, and agree on means to achieve goals (p. 144). Nursing is defined as a process of action, reaction, and interaction whereby nurse and client share information about their perceptions in the nursing situation (p. 2). The goal of nursing is to help individuals maintain their health so they can function in their roles (p.3). 3. *Health:* Health is the dynamic life experiences of a human being, which implies continuous adjustment to stressors in the internal and external	1. If perceptual accuracy is present in nurse-client interactions, transactions will occur. 2. If nurse and client make transactions, goals will be attained. 3. If goals are attained, satisfactions will occur. 4. If goals are attained, effective nursing care will occur. 5. If transactions are made in nurse-client interactions, growth and development will be enhanced. 6. If role expectations and role performance as perceived by nurse and client are congruent, transactions will occur. 7. If role conflict is experienced by nurse or client or both, stress in nurse-client interactions will occur. 8. If nurses with special knowledge and skills communicate	1. *Parsimony:* The theory is logical and organized. Definitions are clear and concise. Assumptions, concepts, definitions, and relationship statements are easily identifiable. 2. *Scope:* Very broad since it contains 16 concepts as well as the four elements of the nursing paradigm—nurse, client, health and environment. 3. *Applicability/Generalizability:* Easily applied to the current practice of nursing. King frequently utilizes nursing situations to assist in the definition of the concept as well as offering implications for nursing practice. I can visualize this theory as being applicable in all nursing settings (including that of the newborn and the comatose patient). The theory of goal attainment is a further development of the steps of the nursing process that are widely used throughout nursing practice. The theory has potential generality since it is broad in scope but not yet thoroughly tested. More re-

(continued on next page)

Assumptions	Concepts	Relationship Statements	Evaluation
12. Individuals have a right to knowledge about themselves. 13. Individuals have a right to participate in decisions that influence their life, their health, and their community services. 14. Health professionals have a responsibility to share information that helps individuals make informed decisions about their health care. 15. Individuals have a right to accept or reject health care. 16. Goals of health professionals and goals of recipients of health care may be incongruent.	environment through optimum use of one's resources to achieve maximum potential for daily living (p. 5). 4. *Environment:* An open system exhibiting permeable boundaries permitting an exchange of matter, energy, and information (p. 69). 5. *Interaction:* A process of perception and communication between person and environment and between person and person, represented by verbal and nonverbal behaviors that are goal-directed (p. 145). 6. *Perception:* Each person's representation of reality. It is each person's subjective world of experience (p. 146). 7. *Communication:* A process whereby information is given from one person to another either directly or indirectly. It is the information component of the interactions (p. 146). 8. *Transaction:* An observable behavior of human beings' interaction with their environment. Transactions are viewed as the valuation component of human interactions (p. 147). 9. *Role:* A set of behaviors expected of persons occupying a position in a social system; rules that define rights and obligations in a position; a relationship with one or more individuals interacting in specific situations for a purpose. (p. 147).	appropriate information to clients, mutual goal setting and goal attainment will occur (p. 149). *Hypotheses:* 1. Perceptual accuracy in nurse-patient interactions increases mutual goal setting. 2. Communication increases mutual goal setting between nurses and patients and leads to satisfactions. 3. Satisfactions in nurses and patients increase goal attainment. 4. Goal attainment decreases stress and anxiety in nursing situations. 5. Goal attainment increases patient learning and coping ability in nursing situations. 6. Role conflict experienced by patients, nurses, or both, decreases transactions in nurse-patient interactions. 7. Congruence in role expectations and role performance increases transactions in nurse-patient interactions (p. 156).	search can be done to validate all aspects of the theory. 4. *Agreement with known data:* This theory is relevant to current practice. It supports King's previous work and builds upon it. 5. *Relevant research:* Graduate students were trained to observe and record nurse-patient interactions. These observations were then analyzed. This study resulted in the classification system used to analyze nurse-patient interactions. Although King gives this example of research, and the methodology in her text, there is room for much more research to test her theory. This testing resulted in the theory of goal attainment at the descriptive level. A classification system was then designed. The theory is useful in practice [Joyce Fitzpatrick and Ann Wahill, *Conceptual Models of Nursing* (Bowie, Md.: Robert J. Brady, 1983), p. 237]. Hypotheses were developed that would provide the groundwork for future research. 6. *Importance to the discipline and profession:* I feel this theory could be utilized by nursing education programs as a model for human interaction. It could be used as a framework for a curriculum. This theory can provide a realistic framework on which to base nursing education, nursing re-

10. *Stress:* A dynamic state whereby a human being interacts with the environment to maintain balance for growth, development, and performance. This involves an exchange of energy and information between the person and the environment for regulation and control of stressors (p. 147).

11. *Growth and Development:* Continuous changes in individuals at the cellular, molecular, and behavioral levels of activities. The processes that take place in the life of individuals that help them move from potential capacity for achievement to self-actualization (p. 148).

12. *Time:* A sequence of events moving onward to the future. Time is a continuous flow of events in successive order that implies change, a past, and a future (p. 148).

13. *Space:* Space is defined as existing in all directions and is the same everywhere. It is the physical area called territory, and is defined by the behavior of individuals occupying space, such as gestures, postures, and visible boundaries erected to mark off personal space (p. 148).

search, and nursing practice. Although the emphasis is on the personal and interpersonal systems, the concepts related to social systems are particularly relevant to nursing administration and other positions of leadership. The hypotheses developed as a result of King's research provide fertile ground for further research.

Appendix H. King's Conceptual Framework for Nursing

Theorist: Imogene M. King

Theory: Conceptual Framework for Nursing (Systems Approach)

Phenomenon Observed: Nursing Practice

Analysis by: Marjorie McCullagh, R.N., B.S.N., graduate student, University of North Dakota

Reference: Imogene King, *A Theory for Nursing* (New York: John Wiley, 1981).

Assumptions	Concepts	Relationship Statements	Evaluation
Re: Human Beings: 1. Individuals are social, sentient, rational, reacting, perceiving, controlling, purposeful, action-oriented, time-oriented. Re: Nurse-client Interactions: 2. Perceptions of nurse and client influence the interaction process. 3. Goals, needs, and values of nurse and client influence the interaction process. 4. Individuals have a right to knowledge about themselves. 5. Individuals have a right to participate in decisions that influence their life, their health, and their community services. 6. Health professionals have a responsibility to share information that helps individuals make informed decisions about their health care. 7. Individuals have a right to accept or to reject health care. 8. Goals of health professionals	1. *Nursing* (p. 2): Process of action, reaction, and interaction whereby nurse and client share information about their perceptions in the nursing situation. 2. *Health* (p. 4): Dynamic life experiences of a human being, which implies continuous adjustment to stressors in the internal and external environment through optimum use of one's resources to achieve maximum potential for daily living. 3. *Perception* (p. 146): Each person's representation of reality. Includes: a. Import of energy from environment organized by information b. Transformation of energy by information c. Processing of information d. Sorting of information e. Export of information in overt behavior 4. *Self* (p. 26–27): Composite of thoughts and feelings which constitute a person's awareness of his individual existence, his conception of who and what he is. Constitutes a person's inner world as distinguished	1. If perceptual accuracy is present in nurse-client interactions, transactions will occur. 2. If nurse and client make transactions, goals will be attained. 3. If goals are attained, satisfactions will occur. 4. If goals are attained, effective nursing care will occur. 5. If transactions are made in nurse-client interactions, growth and development will be enhanced. 6. If role expectations and role performance as perceived by nurse and client are congruent, transactions will occur. 7. If role conflict is experienced by nurse or client or both, stress in nurse-client interactions will occur. 8. If nurses with special knowledge and skills communicate appropriate information to clients, mutual goal setting and goal attainment will occur.	1. *Parsimony:* This theory includes multiple concepts to learn, and somewhat fewer assumptions and relationship statements. Some terminology is not defined; for example, "reacting beings" and "controlling beings." Some definitions of concepts are based on the stress adaptation model and systems theory, knowledge of which would be helpful. Is concisely stated in one text. 2. *Scope:* Addresses wide scope of nursing practice. Does not provide for some current nursing functions. Nursing functions are primarily based on "perceptions" and "transactions." Lacks reference to the multi-dimensional aspects of humans (physiological and spiritual). 3. *Applicability and generalizability:* Seems widely applicable to nursing in many areas, especially where teaching and counseling functions are addressed. Less applicable in physiological and spiritual aspects. "Transactions" dependent on client's ability to develop perceptions and agree on goals, means to achieve goals, move

and goals of recipients of health care may be incongruent.

9. Generally, patients and nurses communicate information, mutually set goals, and take action to attain goals.

from the outer world consisting of all people and things.

5. *Man* (p. 143): A social, sentient, rational, reacting, perceiving, controlling, purposeful, action-oriented, time-oriented being.

6. *Human interactions* (p. 59): A process of perception and communication between person and environment and between person and person, represented by verbal and nonverbal behaviors that are goal-directed.

7. *Communication* (p. 146): A process whereby information is given from one person to another directly or indirectly.

8. *Transactions* (p. 147): The valuation component of human interactions; involves bargaining, negotiating, and social exchange.

9. *Role* (p. 147): A set of behaviors expected of persons occupying a position in a social system; rules that define rights and obligations in a position; a relationship with one or more individuals interacting in specific situations for a purpose.

10. *Stress* (p. 147): A dynamic state whereby a human being interacts with the environment to maintain balance for growth, development and performance.

11. *Environment*: An open system exhibiting permeable boundaries permitting an exchange of matter, energy, and information with human beings.

toward goals. (Note also that goals stated as examples are stated in terms of nurse, and may be confused with approaches.)

4. *Agreement with known data*: Compatible with accepted nursing frameworks as well as with many theories borrowed from psychology and sociology. Allows room for development of theory into physiological and spiritual areas. Incomplete. Potentially generalizable to diverse nursing functions.

5. *Relevant Research*: Author describes a study conducted to explain nurse-client interactions that lead to transactions.

6. *Importance to the discipline and profession*: Presents relationship statements that may provide a helpful framework for organizing and researching nursing science in psychosocial and educational domains. Less helpful in physiological and spiritual aspects. Does not present new information but suggests a way of organizing known information and new information for nurses. Places role of client on similar level as nurse in responsibility in achieving goals. Explores reciprocal relationship of client and nurse and how interactions may produce changes in nurse as well as client. Is process-oriented.

Author Index

Subject Index

Acknowledgments

Figures 4, 5, and 6: From Kim Giffin and Bobby R. Patton, *Personal Communication in Human Relations* (Columbus, OH: Merrill, 1974). Reprinted by permission.

Figure 10: Reprinted by permission of Ingeborg G. Mauksch, Ph.D., F.A.A.N., Lecturer and Consultant in Nursing.

Figures 18 and 20: Adapted from B. W. Duldt et al., *Participant's Manual for Anger Workshops* (Minneapolis, MN: Metropolitan Medical Center, 1983). Reprinted by permission.

Chapter 1 draws on material presented in Bonnie Weaver Duldt, Kim Giffin, and Bobby R. Patton, *Interpersonal Communication in Nursing: A Humanistic Approach* (Philadelphia: F. A. Davis, 1983).

Appendix B: Quotations from Sister Callista Roy and Sharon L. Roberts, *Theory Construction in Nursing: An Adaptation Model* (Englewood Cliffs, NJ: Prentice-Hall, 1981) are reprinted by permission of the publisher.

Appendix C: Quotations from Bonnie Weaver Duldt, Kim Giffin, and Bobby R. Patton, *Interpersonal Communication in Nursing: A Humanistic Approach* (Philadelphia: F. A. Davis, 1983) are reprinted by permission of the publisher.

Appendix D: Quotations from Margaret A. Newman, *Theory Development in Nursing* (Philadelphia: F. A. Davis, 1979) are reprinted by permission of the publisher.

Appendix E and Appendix F: Quotations from Jean Watson, *Nursing: The Philosophy and Science of Caring* (Boston: Little, Brown, 1979) are reprinted by permission of the author.

Appendix G and Appendix H: Quotations from Imogene M. King, *A Theory for Nursing: Systems, Concepts and Process*, copyright © 1981 by John Wiley & Sons, Inc., are reprinted by permission of the publisher.

DATE DUE

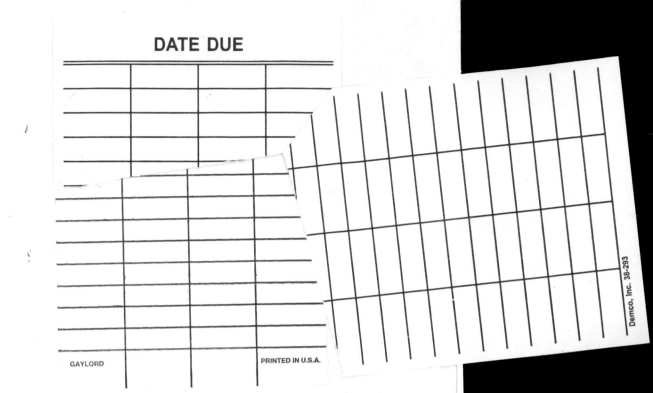

GAYLORD

PRINTED IN U.S.A.

Demco, Inc. 38-293